ANTIBIOTICS
SIMP

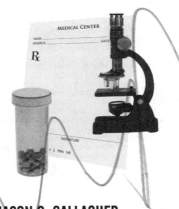

JASON C. GALLAGHER, PHARMD, BCPS
ASSISTANT PROFESSOR OF PHARMACY
TEMPLE UNIVERSITY SCHOOL OF PHARMACY
ADJUNCT ASSISTANT PROFESSOR OF PHARMACOLOGY AND PHYSIOLOGY
DREXEL UNIVERSITY SCHOOL OF MEDICINE

CONAN MacDOUGALL, PHARMD, BCPS
ASSISTANT PROFESSOR OF CLINICAL PHARMACY
UNIVERSITY OF CALIFORNIA, SAN FRANCISCO SCHOOL OF PHARMACY

JONES AND BARTLETT PUBLISHERS
Sudbury, Massachusetts
BOSTON   TORONTO   LONDON   SINGAPORE

World Headquarters

Jones and Bartlett Publishers
40 Tall Pine Drive
Sudbury, MA 01776
978-443-5000
info@jbpub.com
www.jbpub.com

Jones and Bartlett
Publishers Canada
6339 Ormindale Way
Mississauga, Ontario L5V 1J2
Canada

Jones and Bartlett
Publishers International
Barb House, Barb Mews
London W6 7PA
United Kingdom

Jones and Bartlett's books and products are available through most bookstores and online booksellers. To contact Jones and Bartlett Publishers directly, call 800-832-0034, fax 978-443-8000, or visit our website www.jbpub.com.

Substantial discounts on bulk quantities of Jones and Bartlett's publications are available to corporations, professional associations, and other qualified organizations. For details and specific discount information, contact the special sales department at Jones and Bartlett via the above contact information or send an email to specialsales@jbpub.com

The authors and publisher have made every effort to provide accurate information. However, they are not responsible for errors, omissions, or for any outcomes related to the use of the contents of this book and take no responsibility for the use of the products and procedures described. Treatments and side effects described in this book may not be applicable to all people; likewise, some people may require a dose or experience a side effect that is not described herein. Drugs and medical devices are discussed that may have limited availability controlled by the Food and Drug Administration (FDA) for use only in a research study or clinical trial. Research, clinical practice, and government regulations often change the accepted standard in this field. When consideration is being given to use of any drug in the clinical setting, the health care provider or reader is responsible for determining FDA status of the drug, reading the package insert, and reviewing prescribing information for the most up-to-date recommendations on dose, precautions, and contraindications, and determining the appropriate usage for the product. This is especially important in the case of drugs that are new or seldom used.

Production Credits
Executive Editor: David Cella
Acquisitions Editor: Kristine Johnson
Editorial Assistant: Maro Asadoorian
Associate Marketing Manager:
  Lisa Gordon
Production Director: Amy Rose
Senior Production Editor: Susan Schultz

Manufacturing and Inventory Control
  Supervisor: Amy Bacus
Composition: Modern Graphics
Cover Design: Brian Moore
Cover Image: © Photos.com; © The Supe87/
  ShutterShock, Inc.; © Able Stock
Printing and Binding: Malloy, Inc.
Cover Printing: Malloy, Inc.

Library of Congress Cataloging-in-Publication Data

Gallagher, Jason C.
  Antibiotics, simplified / Jason C. Gallagher, Conan MacDougall.
    p. cm.
  ISBN 978-0-7637-5959-9 (pbk.)
  1. Antibiotics. I. MacDougall, Conan. II. Title.
  [DNLM: 1. Anti-Bacterial Agents. QV 350 G162a 2009]
  RM267.G27 2009
  615'.7922—dc22

                                              2008011435

6048

Printed in the United States of America

12 11 10 09 08   10 9 8 7 6 5 4 3 2 1

Contents

Acknowledgments

Our thanks go to those who helped to edit this text, and to our wives who put up with us while we wrote it.

We dedicate this text to the pharmacy students of Temple University and University of California, San Francisco. We hope you find it useful.

Introduction

Antibiotics—the word sends terror coursing through the veins of students and makes many healthcare professionals uncomfortable. The category of antibiotics actually contains many different classes of drugs that differ in spectrum of activity, adverse effect profiles, pharmacokinetics and pharmacodynamics, and clinical utility. These classes can seem bewildering and beyond comprehension. We believe that taking a logical, stepwise approach to learning the pharmacotherapy of infectious diseases can help burn away the mental fog preventing optimal use of these drugs.

Learning the characteristics of antibiotics simplifies learning infectious disease pharmacotherapy. Students and clinicians who attempt to learn the antibiotics of choice for different types of infections before knowing the characteristics of those drugs never truly understand the context of what they are attempting to learn. Once the characteristics of the antibiotics are known, making a logical choice to treat an infection is much easier. This approach takes some time up front, but it will be well worth the effort when the clinician realizes that the pharmacotherapy of all infections is fundamentally similar and logical.

▓ How to Use This Book

We wrote this book in an effort to condense the many facts that are taught about antibiotics in pharmacology courses into one quick reference guide. It is meant to *supplement* material learned in pharmacology, not *supplant* it. Use this book as a reference when you encounter a class of antibiotics that you know you heard about, but may have forgotten key points that impress clinicians and faculty alike.

This book contains three parts. Part 1 reviews basic microbiology and how to approach the pharmacotherapy of a patient with a presumed infection. The chapters in Parts 2 and 3 that follow contain concise reviews of various classes of antibacterial drugs and antifungal drugs, respectively. Again, these are not meant to replace facts learned in pharmacology, but to supplement them. These chapters consist of key points for each class of antibiotics—they are not thorough reviews.

▓ Format of the Drug Class Reviews

Each drug class chapter follows the same basic format. The agents belonging to each class are listed first. The drugs used most commonly in practice are **bolded**.

Spectrum of Activity

The spectra listed are not exhaustive, but only summarize *key organisms* against which each class has or does not have activity.

Adverse Effects

This section lists *key* adverse effects. This list is not exhaustive, but mentions the most common and/or concerning adverse effects of each class.

Dosing Issues

For select drug classes, we include this section to identify common problems or potential errors in drug dosing.

Important Points

This is a summary of significant facts for each drug class.

What They're Good For

This lists some of the most common and/or useful indications for the agents in the class. Many of them are not indicated by the United States Food and Drug Administration (FDA) for these uses, but they are used for them regardless. Conversely, many FDA indications that the antibiotics have will not be listed here.

Don't Forget!

Here we list points that are often overlooked or especially important when dealing with the drug class.

As you move through this book, try to think of situations where the antibiotics would be useful to you. Think of *why* an antibiotic is useful for an indication; don't just learn *that* it is. It is our sincere hope that you too have that magic moment where the world of antibiotics and the study of infectious diseases click together. Let us know when it happens.

Considerations with Antibiotic Therapy

PART 1

The Wonderful World of Microbiology

Despite the promises of the household-products industry, almost *every surface* is covered in microorganisms almost *all the time*. Swab a countertop, your skin, or your dinner and you will find a little world—and that only covers the estimated 10% of bacteria that can be cultured! Obviously, trying to sterilize our patients (and our countertops) is futile; we have to try to target the bad bacteria and let the rest happily crawl all over us. See Appendix 1 for an illustration of how "not clean" we are.

In the microbial world, bacteria lie toward the "less like us" end of the spectrum (**Figure 1-1**). They are prokaryotes, not eukaryotes like fungi, protozoa, and humans. Differences between bacterial and human cells in their anatomy, biochemistry, and the selectivity of antibiotic targets is what allows for the safe and efficacious use of antibiotics.

Differentiating bacteria that are responsible for infection from those just along for the ride can be difficult. Many bacteria that can cause human disease are also normal commensal flora, including *Escherichia coli*, *Streptococcus pneumoniae*, and *Staphylococcus aureus*. Thus, growth of one of these organisms from a culture is not necessarily synonymous with infection. Suspicion of infection is increased greatly if the organism grows from a

Less like us

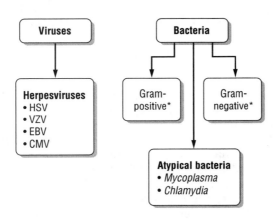

*See Figure 1-2

Figure 1-1
The Microbial World

normally sterile site, such as the bloodstream or cerebrospinal fluid (CSF). Indicators of infection in nonsterile sites (such as sputum and wound cultures) are a high number of organisms, presence of inflammatory cells, and symptoms referable to the culture site (e.g., cough or dyspnea in a patient with a sputum culture growing *S. pneumoniae*, redness and pain in a patient with a skin culture growing *S. aureus*).

Definitive identification and susceptibility testing may take hours to months, depending on the organism and the methods used. Microscopic exam-

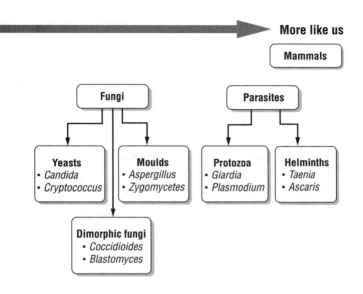

ination and staining may allow for rapid preliminary identification. For bacteria, the most important of these techniques is the Gram's stain. Being able to interpret preliminary microbiology results will allow you to provide the most appropriate therapy to your patients as early as possible.

One of the most fundamental differences among types of bacteria is how they react to a Gram's stain. Gram's stain (crystal violet) is a substance that selectively stains the cell walls of Gram-positive bacteria but is easily washed away from Gram-negative bacteria. Why? In Gram-positive

bacteria, the outermost layer is a thick layer of peptidoglycan, a cellular substance that gives bacterial
cells rigidity. In contrast, Gram-negative bacteria
have an outer membrane of lipopolysaccharides that
blocks the stain from adhering to the peptidoglycan
within the cell (Figure 1-2). Gram-negatives also contain peptidoglycan, but in smaller amounts, and it
is not the outermost layer of the cell. Both Gram-
positive and Gram-negative organisms contain an
inner cell membrane that separates the cell wall
from the cytoplasm of the organism.

Figures 1-3 and 1-4 diagram how you can identify
different bacteria by differences in morphology,
oxygen tolerance, and biochemical identification.

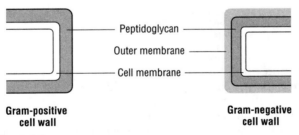

Gram-positive   **Gram-negative**
cell wall   **cell wall**

Figure 1-2
Cell Walls of Gram-Positive and Gram-Negative Organisms

Figure 1-3
Gram-Positive Bacteria

Rapid identification of Gram-positive bacteria based on morphology and preliminary biochemical tests can help to direct therapy.

1. **Morphology:** Most medically important Gram-positive pathogens are cocci (spheres) rather than bacilli (rods). The finding of Gram-positive bacilli should be interpreted within the clinical context: in blood cultures, Gram-positive bacilli often represent common skin contaminants (such as *Propionibacterium*, *Corynebacterium*, and *Bacillus* species). Detection of Gram-positive bacilli from necrotizing wound infections suggests clostridial infection, whereas the finding of Gram-positive bacilli in CSF cultures raises the concern for *Listeria*.

2. **Colony clustering:** Within the Gram-positive cocci, the staphylococci tend to form clusters, whereas the streptococci (including enterococci) typically appear in pairs or chains. The rapid catalase test also helps to differentiate staphylococci from streptococci. Again, the clinical context aids in interpretation: The finding of streptococci in a respiratory culture suggests *S. pneumoniae*, while a report of "streptococci" from an intra-abdominal culture suggests *Enterococcus* (which may be identified preliminarily as a *Streptococcus*).

3. **Biochemistry and appearance on agar:** The coagulase test is useful for differentiating the more virulent (coagulase-positive) *S. aureus* from its cousin the coagulase-negative *S. epidermidis*. *S. epidermidis* is a frequent contaminant of blood cultures; if only one of a pair of blood samples is positive for coagulase-negative staphylococci, treatment may not be required. The pattern of hemolysis (clearing around colonies on agar plates) helps to differentiate among the streptococci: the oral flora (α-hemolytic *S. pneumoniae* and the viridans strep), pathogens of the skin, pharynx, and genitourinary tract (β-hemolytic Group A and B strep), and the bugs of gastrointestinal origin (non-hemolytic enterococci: the more common *E. faecalis* and the more resistant *E. faecium*).

(continues)

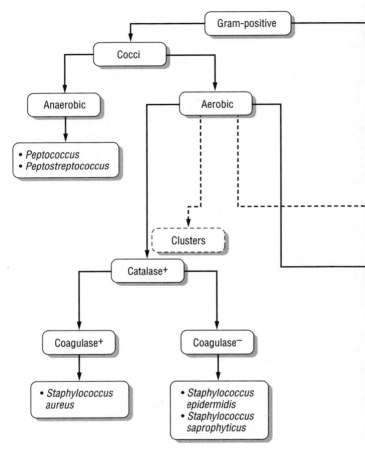

Figure 1-3
Gram-Positive Bacteria *(continued)*

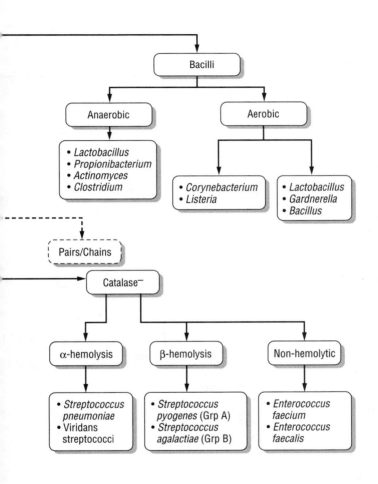

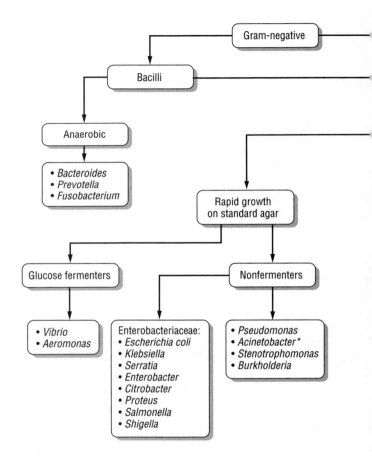

Figure 1-4
Gram-Negative Bacteria

Preliminary identification is somewhat less useful with the Gram-negative bacteria as more extensive biochemical tests are usually needed to differentiate among them.

1. **Morphology:** Among Gram-negative pathogens, the bacilli predominate. The situation in which identification of Gram-negative

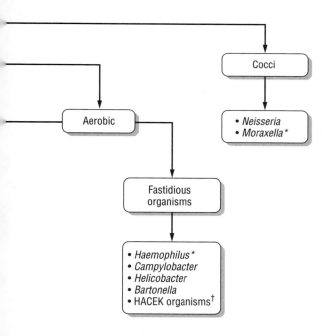

* = these organisms may appear as coccobacilli
† = *Haemophilus, Actinobacillus, Cardiobacterium, Eikenella, Kingella*

cocci would be most useful is in the setting of meningitis, where this
finding would strongly suggest *Neisseria meningitidis*. Note also that
some organisms have a characteristic "coccobacillary" appearance,
which may suggest *H. influenzae*, *Moraxella*, or *Acinetobacter*.

2. **Glucose/lactose fermentation:** The pathogens within the family
Enterobacteriaceae (including *E. coli*, *Klebsiella*, *Serratia*, *Proteus*,
and *Enterobacter*) generally ferment glucose/lactose; at this point

(continues)

Figure 1-4
Gram-Negative Bacteria *(continued)*

the lab may identify them as "enteric Gram-negative rods." In contrast, *Pseudomonas*, *Acinetobacter*, *Stenotrophomonas*, and *Burkholderia* are "nonfermenters;" a report of "nonfermenting Gram-negative rods" should lead you to reassess and if necessary broaden your antibiotic coverage, since these organisms have in common a high level of antibiotic resistance.

3. **Fastidious organisms:** These organisms are picky eaters—they grow slowly and often require specially supplemented media. Thus, it may take a few days to a few weeks for them to grow from culture.

General Approach to Infectious Diseases

2

The pharmacotherapy of infectious diseases confuses many clinicians, but the approach to the patient with an infection is relatively simple and consistent. Understanding this approach is the first step in developing a useful expertise in infectious diseases and antibiotic use.

Prophylactic Therapy

The use of antimicrobial chemotherapy—that is, the treatment of microorganisms with chemical agents—falls into one of three general categories: prophylaxis, empiric use, and definitive therapy. *Prophylaxis* is treatment given to prevent an infection that has not yet developed. Use of prophylactic therapy is limited to patients at high risk of complications from an infection, such as those on immunosuppressive therapy, those with cancer, or patients who are having surgery. These patients have weakened natural defenses that render them susceptible to infection. Because the likelihood of infection by some types of organisms in these patients is high and the consequences of infection are dire, we administer antimicrobial drugs to prevent infections from occurring. However, the world is not sterile and breakthrough infections do occur. The key to understanding antimicrobial prophylaxis is to remember that patients who receive it do not have an infection, but are at risk for one.

Empiric Therapy

Unlike prophylactic therapy, *empiric therapy* is given to patients who have a proven or suspected infection, but the responsible organism(s) has or have not yet been identified. It is the type of therapy most often initiated in both outpatient and inpatient settings. After the clinician assesses the likelihood of an infection based on physical exam, laboratory findings, and other signs and symptoms, s/he usually will collect samples for culture and Gram staining. For most types of cultures, the Gram stain is performed relatively quickly. In the Gram stain, details about the site of infection are revealed, such as the presence of organisms and white blood cells (WBCs), morphology of the organisms present (e.g., Gram-positive cocci in clusters), and the nature of the sample itself, which in some cases describes if the sample is adequate. The process of culturing the sample begins around the time that the clinician performs the Gram stain. After a day or so, biochemical testing will reveal the identification of the organism, and eventually the organism will be tested for its susceptibility to various antibiotics.

However, this process takes several days, so empiric therapy is initiated *before* the clinician knows the exact identification and susceptibilities of the causative organism. Empiric therapy is our best guess of which antimicrobial agent or agents will be most active against the likely cause of infection. Sometimes we are right, and sometimes we are wrong. Keep in mind that empiric therapy should not be directed against every known organism in nature, just those most likely to cause the infection in question.

Definitive Therapy

After culture and sensitivity results are known, the *definitive therapy* phase of treatment can begin. Unlike empiric therapy, with definitive therapy we know on what organisms to base our treatment and which drugs should work against them. At this phase it is prudent to choose antimicrobial agents that are safe, effective, narrow in spectrum, and cost effective. This helps us avoid unneeded toxicity, treatment failures, and the possible emergence of antimicrobial resistance and it also helps manage costs. In general, moving from empiric to definitive therapy involves decreasing coverage, because we do not need to target organisms that are not causing infection in our patient. In fact, giving overly broad-spectrum antibiotics can lead to the development of superinfections, infections caused by organisms resistant to the antibiotics in use that occur during therapy.

The clinician who is treating an infected patient should strive to make the transition to definitive therapy. Although it seems obvious, this does not always occur. If the patient improves on the first antibiotic, clinicians may be reluctant to transition to more narrow-spectrum therapy. Also, some infections may resolve with empiric therapy before culture results would even be available, such as uncomplicated urinary tract infections. In other cases, cultures may not be obtained or may be negative in spite of strong signs that the patient has an infection (e.g., clinical symptoms, fever, increased WBC count). In most situations it is important that clinicians continuously consider the need to transition to definitive therapy. Overly broad-spectrum therapy has consequences and the next infection is likely to be harder to treat. Keep in mind the general pathway for the treatment of infectious diseases shown in **Figure 2-1**.

Examples of Therapy

Here are a few examples of each type of therapy:

Prophylaxis

- Trimethoprim-sulfamethoxazole to prevent *Pneumocystis jirovecii* (formerly *carinii*) pneumonia in a patient on cyclosporine and prednisone after a liver transplant
- Azithromycin to prevent *Mycobacterium avium intracellularae* in an advanced HIV patient
- Cefazolin given before surgery to prevent a staphylococcal skin infection of the surgical site

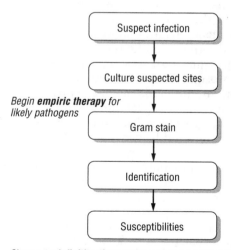

*Change to **definitive therapy** for patient-specific pathogens*

Figure 2-1
General Approach to Infectious Diseases

Empiric therapy

- Levofloxacin initiated for a patient with pre-sumed community-acquired pneumonia
- Ceftriaxone given for the treatment of suspected pyelonephritis
- Vancomycin, tobramycin, and meropenem for a patient with probable hospital-acquired pneumonia in the intensive care unit

Definitive therapy

- Transitioning from piperacillin/tazobactam to ampicillin in a patient with a wound infection caused by *Enterococcus faecalis* that is susceptible to both drugs
- Discontinuing ceftriaxone and initiating ciprofloxacin for a patient with a urinary tract infection caused by *Klebsiella pneumoniae* that is resistant to ceftriaxone but susceptible to ciprofloxacin
- Narrowing therapy from vancomycin, ciprofloxacin, and imipenem/cilastatin to vancomycin alone for a patient with hospital-acquired pneumonia whose deep respiratory culture grew only methicillin-resistant *Staphylococcus aureus* (MRSA) that is susceptible to vancomycin

Case Study

Here is an example of treating a patient with an infection by the above pathway:

TR is a 63-year-old man with a past medical history of diabetes, hypertension, and coronary artery disease who comes to the hospital complaining of pain, redness and swelling around a wound on his foot. Close inspection reveals that he has an infected diabetic foot ulcer. He is admitted to the hospital (Day 1). The clinician performs surgical debridement that evening and sends cultures from the wound during surgery as well as blood cultures. The clinician initiates *empiric therapy* with vancomycin and piperacillin/tazobactam.

On Day 2, Gram stain results from the wound are available. There are many white blood cells with many Gram-positive cocci but no Gram-negative rods, so the clinician discontinues piperacillin/tazobactam. Blood cultures do not grow any organisms.

The following day (Day 3), culture results from the wound reveal many *Staphylococcus aureus*. Because vancomycin is usually effective against this organism, its use is continued.

On Day 4, susceptibility results from the wound culture return. The *S. aureus* is found to be susceptible to methicillin, oxacillin, cefazolin, piperacillin/tazobactam, clindamycin, trimethoprim/sulfamethoxazole, and vancomycin. It is resistant to penicillin, ampicillin, tetracycline, and levofloxacin. As the isolate from TR's wound is methicillin-susceptible *Staphylococcus aureus* (MSSA), the clinician discontinues vancomycin and initiates *definitive therapy* with oxacillin.

Note how in TR's case we began empiric therapy with a broad-spectrum regimen of vancomycin and piperacillin/tazobactam to cover the Gram-positive and Gram-negative aerobes and anaerobes that tend to cause diabetic foot infections but narrowed that therapy gradually as Gram stain and culture data returned. Eventually we were able to choose a highly effective, narrow-spectrum, inexpensive, and safe choice of definitive therapy that was driven by microbiology results. Both vancomycin and piperacillin/tazobactam were active against TR's *Staphylococcus aureus* as well, but both are broader in spectrum than oxacillin and represent less-ideal choices of therapy.

Antibiotic Pharmacodynamics

3

The term *antibiotic pharmacodynamics* refers to the manner in which antibiotics interact with their target organisms to exert their effects: Does the antibiotic kill the organism or just slow its growth? Is it better to give a high dose of antibiotics all at once or to achieve low concentrations for a long time? Clinicians increasingly recognize such considerations as important in maximizing the success of therapy, especially for difficult-to-treat infections or in immunocompromised patients.

Susceptibility Testing

Typically, one judges the susceptibility of a particular organism to an antibiotic based on the minimum inhibitory concentration (MIC) for the organism-antibiotic combination. The clinician determines the MIC by mixing a standard concentration of the organism that the patient has grown with increasing concentrations of the antibiotic in a broth solution. Classically this was done in test tubes (see **Figure 3-1**), but today it is done more commonly on microdilution plates. The mixture is incubated for about a day, and the clinician examines the tubes or plates (with the naked eye or with a computer) for signs of cloudiness, indicating growth of the organism. The mixture with the lowest concentration of antibiotic where there is no visible growth is deemed to be the MIC. For each organism-antibiotic pair there is a particular cutoff

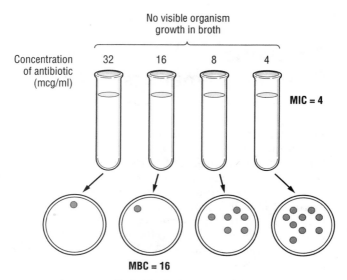

Figure 3-1
Susceptibility Testing of Antibiotics

MIC that is considered susceptible. This particular MIC is called the breakpoint. **Table 3-1** provides examples of breakpoints for different organism/pathogen combinations. Note that just because an antibiotic has the lowest MIC for a pathogen, that does not mean it is the best choice—different antibiotics achieve different concentrations in the body. Thus, antibiotic MICs for a single organism generally should not be compared across different drugs in selecting therapy. Finally, be aware that other methods of susceptibility testing exist, including disk diffusion and E-tests, but that broth dilution methods are generally considered the gold standard.

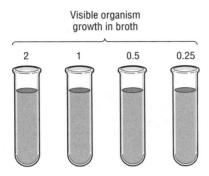

Visible organism growth in broth

| 2 | 1 | 0.5 | 0.25 |

TABLE 3-1

Examples of Antibiotic Susceptibility Breakpoints

Organism Antibiotics	Susceptible	Intermediate	Resistant
E. coli			
Ceftriaxone	≤ 8 mcg/ml	16–32 mcg/ml	≥ 64 mcg/ml
Levofloxacin	≤ 2 mcg/ml	4 mcg/ml	≥ 8 mcg/ml
Trimethoprim/ sulfamethoxazole	≤ 2/38 mcg/ml	—	≥ 4/76 mcg/ml
Streptococcus pneumoniae			
Ceftriaxone*	≤ 0.5 mcg/ml	1 mcg/ml	≥ 2 mcg/ml
Levofloxacin	≤ 2 mcg/ml	4 mcg/ml	≥ 8 mcg/ml
Trimethoprim/ sulfamethoxazole	≤ 0.5/9.5 mcg/ml	1–2/19–38 mcg/ml	≥ 4/76 mcg/ml

*Breakpoint for non-meningeal infections.

Bacteriostatic Versus Bactericidal

At the MIC the antibiotic is inhibiting growth, but it may or may not actually be killing the organism. Antibiotics that inhibit growth of the organism without killing it are termed bacteriostatic. If antibiotics are taken away, the organisms can begin growing again. However, bacteriostatic antibiotics usually are successful in treating infections because they allow the patient's immune system to catch up and kill off the organisms. Other antibiotics are considered bactericidal; their action kills the organisms without any help from the immune system. For most infections, outcomes using appropriate bacteriostatic versus bactericidal drugs are similar; however, for certain infections bactericidal drugs are preferred. These infections include endocarditis, meningitis, osteomyelitis, and infections in neutropenic patients. For these infections, there is reduced contribution from the immune system because of the anatomic location or the immunosuppression of the patient. Bactericidal activity is determined by taking a sample of the broth at the MIC and below and spreading the broth on agar plates (Figure 3-1). The number of bacterial colonies on the plates are counted and the concentration corresponding to a 99.9% reduction in the original bacterial inoculum is considered to be the minimum bactericidal concentration (MBC). When the MBC is 4 times or less the MIC, the drug is considered to be bactericidal; if the MBC/MIC ratio is greater than 4, it is considered bacteriostatic. Table 3-2 lists drugs according to whether they are generally considered bacteriostatic or bactericidal; however, it should be noted that this activity can vary based on the pathogen being treated, the achievable dose, and the growth phase of the organism.

Pharmacokinetic/Pharmacodynamic Relationships

Besides differing in whether they kill bacteria or merely inhibit their growth, antibiotics also differ in how they manifest their effects over time. Careful studies have revealed that for certain antibiotics, activity against bacteria correlates with the duration of time that the concentration of the drug remains above the MIC (time-dependent activity). For other antibiotics, antibacterial activity correlates not with the time above the MIC but with the ratio of the peak concentration of the drug to the MIC (concentration-dependent or time-independent activity). For some antibiotics, the best predictor of activity is the ratio of the area under the concentration-time curve to the MIC. **Figure 3-2** illustrates these pharmacokinetic/pharmacodynamic

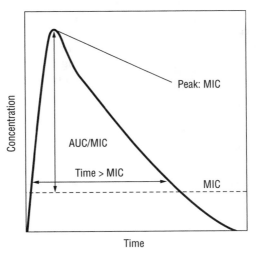

Figure 3-2
Pharmacokinetic/Pharmacodynamic Relationships

(PK/PD) parameters schematically, and Table 3-2 shows which parameter is most predictive of efficacy for antibiotic classes. The practical implications of these findings are in the design of antibiotic dosing schedules: aminoglycosides are now frequently given as a single large dose daily to leverage the con-centration-dependent activity, while some clinicians are administering beta-lactam drugs such as cef-tazidime as continuous infusions because of their time-dependent activity. As target values for these parameters that predict efficacy are found, there may be an increase in the individualization of dosing of antibiotics to achieve these target values.

TABLE 3-2
Antibacterial Activity of Antibiotics

Antibiotic	Antibacterial Activity	Predictive PK/PD Parameter
Penicillins Cephalosporins Carbapenems Monobactams	Bactericidal	Time > MIC
Vancomycin	Bactericidal	AUC/MIC
Fluoroquinolones Aminoglycosides Metronidazole Daptomycin	Bactericidal	Peak:MIC
Macrolides Tetracyclines Clindamycin Linezolid	Bacteriostatic	AUC/MIC

Adverse Consequences of Antibiotic Use

4

Although antibiotics are undoubtedly one of the most beneficial discoveries of science, they are not without risks. They can adversely affect patients by eliciting allergic reactions, causing direct toxicity, or altering the normal bacterial flora, leading to superinfections with other organisms. Antibiotic use is the primary driving force in the development of antibiotic resistance, which can affect not only the treated patients but other patients by transmission of resistant organisms. It is important to keep in mind all of these potential adverse consequences when using antibiotics.

Antibiotic Allergy

Through formation of complexes with human proteins, antibiotics can trigger immunologic reactions. These may manifest immediately (such as anaphylaxis or hives) or be delayed (rashes, serum sickness, drug fever). Because of their highly reactive chemical structure and frequent use, beta-lactam drugs are the most notorious group of drugs for causing allergic reactions. It is difficult to determine how likely it is that a patient with an allergy to a particular antibiotic agent will have a similar reaction to another agent within that class. While some estimates of the degree of cross-reactivity are available for beta-lactam drugs (see below), estimates for cross-reactivity within other classes (for example, between fluoroquinolones) are essentially nonexistent. Because labeling a patient with an allergy to a particular antibiotic can limit future treatment options severely, every effort should be made to clarify the exact nature of a reported allergy.

Antibiotic Toxicities

Despite being designed to affect bacterial rather than human physiology, antibiotics can have direct toxic effects on patients. In some cases this is an extension of their antibacterial mechanism of action: for example, the hematologic adverse effects of trimethoprim stem from its inhibition of folate metabolism in humans. In other cases, antibiotics display toxicity through unintended physiologic interactions, such as when vancomycin stimulates histamine release, leading to its characteristic red man syndrome. Some of these toxicities may be dose related and can be attenuated by dose reduction; this type of toxicity often occurs when doses are not adjusted properly for renal dysfunction.

Superinfection

As Appendix 1 illustrates, the human body is colonized by a variety of different bacteria and fungi. These organisms generally are considered commensals, in that they benefit from living on/in the body but do not cause harm (within their ecologic niches). Colonization with commensal organisms can be beneficial, given that they compete with and crowd out more pathogenic organisms. When administration of antibiotics kills off the commensal flora, pathogenic drug-resistant organisms can flourish due to the absence of competition. This is considered a superinfection (i.e., an infection on top of another infection). For example, administration of antibiotics can lead to the overgrowth of the gastrointestinal pathogen *Clostridium difficile*, which is resistant to most antibiotics. *C. difficile* can cause diarrhea and life-threatening bowel inflammation. Similarly, administration of broad-spectrum antibacterial drugs can select for the overgrowth of fungi, most commonly yeasts of the genus *Candida*. Disseminated *Candida* infections carry a high risk of mortality. To reduce the risk of superinfection, antibiotics should be administered only to patients with proven or probable infections, using the most narrow-spectrum agents appropriate to the infection.

Antibiotic Resistance

Thousands of studies have documented the relationship between antibiotic use and resistance, both at a patient level (if you receive an antibiotic, you are more likely to become infected with a drug-resistant organism) and a society level (the more antibiotics a hospital, region, or country uses, the greater the antibiotic resistance). The development of antibiotic resistance leads to a vicious spiral where resistance necessitates the development of broader-spectrum antibiotics, leading to evolution of bacteria resistant to those new antibiotics, requiring ever broader-spectrum drugs, and so on. This is particularly problematic as antibiotic development has slowed down greatly. Although we can see clearly the broad relationship between antibiotic use and resistance, many of the details of this relationship are not clear. Why do some bacteria develop resistance rapidly and others never develop resistance? What is the proper duration of treatment to maximize the chance of cure and minimize the risk of resistance?

Guidelines

Until we develop a more sophisticated understanding of the relationship between antibiotic use and resistance on a micro level, we are left with some general guidelines for minimizing the potential for development of resistance:

Avoid using antibiotics to treat colonization or contamination.

A substantial percentage of all antibiotic use is directed toward patients who are not truly infected, but in whom organisms are recovered from culture. Isolation of *Staphylococcus epidermidis* from a single blood culture or *Candida* species from a urinary culture in a catheterized patient are common situations in which patients should be scrutinized closely to determine whether an infection is truly present. A proper diagnosis is key.

Use the most narrow-spectrum agent appropriate for the patient's infection.

Broader-spectrum agents multiply the number of bacteria affected by the drug, increasing the chances both for development of resistance and superinfection. "Broader" or "newer" are not synonymous with "better": for example, good old penicillin kills susceptible organisms more rapidly than almost any drug on the market. The treating clinician's goal always should be definitive, narrow-spectrum therapy.

Use the proper dose.

Bacteria that are exposed to low concentrations of antibiotics are more likely to become resistant than those exposed to effective doses. After all, dead bugs don't mutate! Further research in pharmacodynamics should make it easier to determine the proper dose for each patient and thus to reduce the likelihood that resistance will develop.

Use the shortest effective duration of therapy.

Unfortunately, duration of therapy is one of the least-studied areas of infectious diseases. Examination of standard treatment durations says much more about how humans think than about how antibiotics and bacteria truly interact—durations are typically 5, 7, 10, or 14 days, in line with our decimal system and the days in a week. New studies are showing that shorter durations of therapy are just as effective as prolonged courses and possibly less likely to select for resistance. As studies progress and determine additional factors that indicate when infections are sufficiently treated, it should be possible to more accurately define the length of therapy on a patient-by-patient basis.

Antibacterial Drugs

5

Beta-Lactams

■ Introduction to Beta-Lactams

Beta-lactams include a wide variety of antibiotics that seem to exist only to confuse students and clinicians. Penicillins, cephalosporins, and carbapenems are all beta-lactams. Monobactams (aztreonam) are structurally similar, but lack one of the two rings that other beta-lactams have and consequently have little to no cross-allergenicity with other beta-lactams. To make matters more confusing, not all beta-lactams end in -cillin or -penem or start with ceph-.

We believe the best approach to keeping beta-lactams straight is to group them into classes and learn the characteristics of each class. If you work in a hospital, then it is likely that you will have only one or two drugs of each class to worry about. Fortunately, all beta-lactams have a few things in common.

- All beta-lactams can cause hypersensitivity reactions, ranging from mild rashes to drug fever to acute interstitial nephritis to anaphylaxis. There is some cross-sensitivity among classes, but there is no way to predict exactly how often that will occur. Studies on the matter differ greatly in their conclusions.
- Seizures can result from very high doses of any beta-lactam. Some are more notorious for this

adverse effect than others. Did you check your patient's renal function?

- All beta-lactams share a mechanism of action—inhibition of transpeptidases (that is, penicillin-binding proteins) in the bacterial cell wall. Thus, giving two beta-lactams in combination for the same infection generally is not useful. There are a few exceptions to this rule, but not many.
- All beta-lactams lack activity against atypical organisms such as *Mycoplasma pneumoniae* and *Chlamydophila pneumoniae*. Add another drug to your regimen if you are concerned about these bugs, as in community-acquired pneumonia.
- All currently available beta-lactams lack activity against MRSA. Add vancomycin or another agent if this bug is suspected. Newer cephalosporins that are being developed address MRSA, but they are not yet approved by the U.S. Food and Drug Administration (FDA).

Once you know the similarities among beta-lactams, it is easier to learn the differences among them.

Penicillins

■ Introduction to Penicillins

Penicillins are one of the largest and oldest classes of antimicrobial agents. Since the development of the natural penicillins in the 1930s, further penicillin development has been directed by the need to combat increasing antimicrobial resistance. Classes of penicillins with expanded Gram-negative spectra overcome the shortfalls of natural penicillins, and they can be grouped fairly easily by spectrum of activity.

Penicillins have several things in common:

- Penicillins have very short half-lives (<2 hours) and must be dosed multiple times per day. The half-lives of most of them are prolonged in the presence of renal dysfunction.
- Like other beta-lactams, penicillins can cause hypersensitivity reactions. If a patient has a true hypersensitivity reaction to a penicillin, other penicillins should be avoided, even if they are from different classes of penicillins. If the reaction is not severe (that is, not anaphylactoid), cephalosporins and carbapenems may be useful.
- Many penicillins are relatively poorly absorbed, even those available as oral formulations. This can lead to diarrhea when oral

therapy is needed. Pay attention to the dosing of oral versus intravenous penicillins—often, a conversion from intravenous to oral therapy means there will be a substantial decrease in the amount of active drug in the body.

Many penicillins were developed after the natural penicillins became available. Until researchers developed beta-lactamase inhibitors, development primarily focused on *either* improved activity against staphylococci (MSSA) *or* Gram-negative rods (**Figure 5-1**).

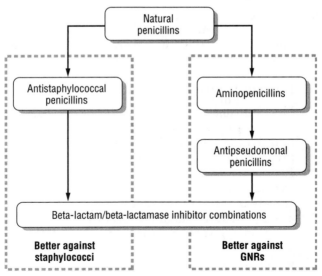

Figure 5-1
Penicillin Drug Development

Natural Penicillins

Agents: penicillin G, penicillin V

All of us have heard of the discovery of penicillin by Sir Alexander Fleming in 1929. Once penicillin was isolated years later, it had a major impact on society, particularly in the treatment of wound infections. The importance of this became apparent during World War II, when the Allies had access to penicillin and the Axis did not. Unfortunately, staphylococci quickly became resistant to penicillin, initiating the search for new beta-lactams and leading to the confusing array of these drugs available today. The development of resistance has narrowed the spectrum of effectiveness of natural penicillins considerably over the past 60 years, such that staphylococci are almost universally resistant to them. Occasionally we still see an isolate of *Staphylococcus aureus* that is susceptible to penicillin.

Spectrum

Good: *Treponema pallidum*, most streptococci
Moderate: *Streptococcus pneumoniae*, enterococci
Poor: almost everything else

Adverse Effects

Similar to adverse effects for other beta-lactams.

▨ Important Facts

- Natural penicillins have a very short half-life and must be dosed frequently or given by continuous infusion. Long-acting depot formulations (procaine, benzathine) are available. It is important to know the differences among these formulations, because the doses vary considerably. It is even more important not to give procaine or benzathine products intravenously, as this can be fatal.
- Penicillin V is the oral form of penicillin G. Other drugs have supplanted it in most, but not all, uses.
- Penicillin G remains the drug of choice for syphilis.
- Due to resistance, penicillin is a poor empiric choice for most infections. Not all medical textbooks have been updated to reflect the changes in penicillin use that have resulted from widespread resistance.

What They're Good For

Syphilis, particularly neurosyphilis. During penicillin shortages, hospitals often reserve its use for this indication. Penicillin is also used in susceptible streptococcal infections such as pharyngitis or endocarditis.

Don't Forget!

Other, more conveniently dosed narrow spectrum beta-lactams are available for bugs treatable with penicillin.

Antistaphylococcal Penicillins

Agents: methicillin, cloxacillin, **dicloxacillin**, **nafcillin**, **oxacillin**

It did not take long for *Staphylococcus* spp. to become resistant to penicillin. Within a few years of penicillin becoming widely available, staphylococcal strains began to produce beta-lactamases, rendering penicillin useless in these infections. The basic structure of penicillin was modified to resist these destructive enzymes, leading to the anti-staphylococcal penicillins. This modification gave these drugs activity against staphylococci that produce penicillinases (beta-lactamases active against penicillins), but did not add to the poor Gram-negative activity of the natural penicillins.

Spectrum
Good: MSSA, streptococci
Poor: Gram-negative rods, enterococci, anaerobes, MRSA

Adverse Effects
Similar to those for other beta-lactams, with a possibly higher incidence of acute interstitial nephritis (AIN).

▨ Important Facts

- Antistaphylococcal penicillins have a short half-life and must be dosed frequently. This presents a problem, because they cause phlebitis. Does your patient have phlebitis? Try a first-generation cephalosporin instead.
- Most are eliminated from the body in large part by the liver and do not need to be adjusted in cases of renal dysfunction.
- These drugs are interchangeable therapeutically. Therefore, *Staphylococcus aureus* that is susceptible to methicillin (which is no longer used) is susceptible to oxacillin, nafcillin, and the rest. That is, MSSA = OSSA = NSSA, etc.

What They're Good For

Infections caused by MSSA, such as endocarditis and skin and soft tissue infections.

Don't Forget!

Beta-lactams kill staphylococci more quickly than vancomycin, so patients with MSSA infections who lack serious beta-lactam allergies should be switched to beta-lactams, such as antistaphylococcal penicillins.

Aminopenicillins

Agents: amoxicillin, ampicillin

Though the antistaphylococcal penicillins improve on the Gram-positive coverage of natural penicillins, they do not add to their Gram-negative coverage. Aminopenicillins are more water-soluble and pass through porin channels in the cell wall of some Gram-negative organisms. However, they are susceptible to beta-lactamases, and resistance to them has become fairly common in many institutions. Aminopenicillins are rarely active against staphylococci, because these produce penicillinase. Also, remember that these drugs do not have useful activity against *Pseudomonas aeruginosa*.

Spectrum
Good: streptococci, enterococci
Moderate: enteric Gram-negative rods, *Haemophilus*
Poor: staphylococci, anaerobes

Adverse Effects
Similar to other beta-lactams. They have a high incidence of diarrhea when given orally.

▨ Important Facts

- Though ampicillin can be given orally, amoxicillin is a better choice. It is more bioavailable, better tolerated, and administered less frequently. Use ampicillin for intravenous therapy, and amoxicillin for oral therapy. Europeans disagree; they use amoxicillin intravenously also.
- Ampicillin is a drug of choice for susceptible enterococci.

What They're Good For

Infections caused by susceptible Gram-negative rods, enterococci, and streptococci. Because resistance among Gram-negative rods is prevalent, aminopenicillins are used only infrequently in complicated nosocomial infections. Amoxicillin frequently is prescribed for infections of the upper respiratory tract, including streptococcal pharyngitis (strep throat) and otitis media (ear infection).

Don't Forget!

To achieve bactericidal activity against enterococci, ampicillin (or any other beta-lactam) has to be combined with an aminoglycoside. This should be done in serious infections such as endocarditis.

Antipseudomonal Penicillins

Agents: piperacillin, mezlocillin, carbenicillin, **ticarcillin**

None of the penicillins we have discussed thus far offer appreciable activity against *Pseudomonas aeruginosa*, a common nosocomial pathogen that is often resistant to multiple antibiotics. Enter the antipseudomonal penicillins. These agents are active against *Pseudomonas aeruginosa* and other more drug-resistant Gram-negative rods. However, they are just as susceptible to beta-lactamases as penicillin and ampicillin, so they are not anti-staphylococcal. Also, strains of Gram-negative rods that produce beta-lactamases are resistant to them. They do have activity against streptococci and enterococci.

Spectrum

Good: *Pseudomonas aeruginosa*, streptococci, enterococci

Moderate: enteric Gram-negative rods, *Haemophilus*

Poor: staphylococci, anaerobes

Adverse Effects

Similar to other beta-lactams.

▇ Important Facts
- These drugs retain the Gram-positive activity of penicillin and are active against many streptococci and enterococci.
- Antipseudomonal penicillins can be used by themselves or, more commonly, in combination with a beta-lactamase inhibitor (see the next section).
- Piperacillin is the most frequently prescribed of these agents. It has stronger antipseudomonal activity than ticarcillin. Carbenicillin is oral, but does not achieve useful concentrations for the treatment of anything except urinary tract infections. Mezlocillin is not commonly used.

What They're Good For
Infections caused by susceptible *Pseudomonas* or other Gram-negative rods. If a Gram-positive organism is susceptible to an antipseudomonal penicillin, it will be susceptible to narrow-spectrum penicillins as well, and the narrower-spectrum drug should be used.

Don't Forget!
These drugs are useful step-down agents in the treatment of infections caused by *Pseudomonas aeruginosa*. However, they are not good empiric therapeutic choices, because other Gram-negative rods that cause nosocomial infections may be resistant to them (such as *E. coli*). Start with a beta-lactamase-resistant agent, then change your therapy to an antipseudomonal penicillin if susceptibilities allow.

Beta-Lactam/Beta-Lactamase Inhibitor Combinations

Agents: ampicillin/sulbactam, amoxicillin/ clavulanate, ticarcillin/clavulanate, piperacillin/tazobactam

Though the aminopenicillins and antipseudomonal penicillins have good intrinsic activity against Gram-negative rods, they remain just as susceptible to beta-lactamases as penicillin G. This means that they are not useful against staphylococci or many Gram-negative rods and anaerobes, because these organisms have learned to produce beta-lactamase. In other words, it seemed we learned how to either make a penicillin resistant to beta-lactamase, or how to make it more active against Gram-negative rods, but not both. Beta-lactamase inhibitors counter beta-lactamases; these drugs mimic the structure of beta-lactams but have little antimicrobial activity on their own. They bind to beta-lactamases irreversibly, preventing the beta-lactamase from destroying any beta-lactams that are co-administered and enabling therapeutic beta-lactam to be effective.

When considering the activity of the beta-lactam/beta-lactamase inhibitor combination, remember that the beta-lactamase inhibitor only frees up the beta-lactam to kill the organism—it doesn't enhance the activity. Therefore, the combination products are only active against the bacteria that the beta-lactam in the combination has intrinsic activity against. For example, ampicillin/sulbactam is active against beta-lactamase producing *E. coli,* because ampicillin alone is active against non-beta-lactamase producing *E. coli*. However, it has no useful activity against *Pseudomonas aeruginosa* because ampicillin lacks activity against this organism. On the other hand, piperacillin/tazobactam is active against *P. aeruginosa* because piperacillin alone is useful. Though these drugs have very broad spectra of activity, there are differences among the agents. Keep this rule in mind to set them straight.

Spectrum

Good: MSSA, streptococci, enterococci, many anaerobes, enteric GNRs, *Pseudomonas aeruginosa* (only piperacillin/tazobactam and ticarcillin/clavulanate)

Moderate: Gram-negative rods with advanced beta-lactamases

Poor: MRSA, extended-spectrum beta-lactamase (ESBL) producing GNRs

Adverse Effects

Similar to other beta-lactams.

Important Facts

- Unlike the other members of this class, amoxicillin/clavulanate is available orally. Various doses are available, but higher ones are associated with more diarrhea.

- The beta-lactamase inhibitors packaged in these combinations are not active against all beta-lactamases. New beta-lactamases with the ability to destroy many types of beta-lactams are continually being discovered and are becoming more prevalent.

- Except for study purposes, beta-lactamase inhibitors are not available outside of the combination products.
- Sulbactam has good activity against *Acinetobacter baumanni*, a highly drug-resistant Gram-negative rod that causes nosocomial infections. For this reason, high doses of ampicillin/sulbactam can be used in the treatment of infections caused by this organism.

What They're Good For

Empiric therapy of nosocomial infections, particularly nosocomial pneumonia (not aminopenicillin-based combinations). Because they have activity against aerobes and anaerobes, they are a good empiric choice for mixed infections, such as intra-abdominal infections, diabetic ulcers, and aspiration pneumonia.

Don't Forget!

Narrow your coverage once culture results return. These are good choices of empiric therapy, but poor choices of definitive therapy if alternatives are available. Be sure you know which drugs are antipseudomonal and which are not—this is a major difference among these agents that drives their use. Ampicillin/sulbactam is a poor choice for nosocomial pneumonia, and piperacillin/tazobactam is overkill for community-acquired pneumonia.

Cephalosporins

Introduction to Cephalosporins

The cephalosporins are probably the most confusing group of antibiotics. For convenience, they have been grouped into "generations" that largely correlate with their spectrum of activity, with some notable exceptions. Although there are many different individual agents, the good news is that most hospitals only use a few of them, so, in practice, learning your institution's cephalosporins of choice is easy. In general, it is best to learn the characteristics of each generation and then learn the quirks about the individual agents.

Cephalosporins have several elements in common:

- All have reduced cross-allergenicity with penicillins, though there are differences among generations. Estimates about the likelihood of cross-reactivity between penicillin and cephalosporin allergies differ. It is likely very low, below the oft-quoted 10%. A reasonable estimate is no more than 3% to 5%, though some publications support even lower numbers, particularly for later-generation agents. However, using any cephalosporin in a patient with a penicillin allergy is a matter of balancing risks and benefits. Assess the validity of the patient's allergy through interview and consider the level of risk associated with cephalosporin administration. Be skeptical of nausea, but be sure to take hives and any signs of anaphylaxis *very* seriously! Always use alternative classes of antibiotics when practical.

- The cephalosporins are generally more resistant to beta-lactamases than penicillins are. Beta-lactamases that are active against penicillins but inactive against cephalosporins are called *penicillinases*. Beta-lactamases that inactivate cephalosporins (*cephalosporinases*) also exist.

- None of the cephalosporins have useful activity against enterococci.

First-Generation Cephalosporins

Agents: cefazolin, **cephalexin**, cefadroxil, cephalothin

First-generation cephalosporins are the most commonly used class of antibiotics in the hospital. Why? They are used immediately prior to surgery to prevent surgical site infections. Their spectrum of activity, inexpensive cost, and low incidence of adverse effects make them ideal for this purpose.

Spectrum
Good: MSSA, streptococci
Moderate: some enteric Gram-negative rods
Poor: enterococci, anaerobes, MRSA, *Pseudomonas*

Adverse Effects
Similar to other beta-lactams.

■ Important Facts
- First-generation cephalosporins are good alternatives to antistaphylococcal penicillins. They cause less phlebitis and are infused less frequently. Unlike antistaphylococcal penicillins, however, they do not cross the blood-brain barrier and should not be used in central nervous system (CNS) infections.

- Cephalexin and cefadroxil are available orally; the others are parenteral.

What They're Good For

Skin and soft tissue infections, surgical prophylaxis, staphylococcal endocarditis (MSSA).

Don't Forget!

Surgical prophylaxis is the most common indication for first-generation cephalosporins in the hospital. Be sure to limit the duration of therapy for this use; administering more than one dose of antibiotics should be uncommon, and giving more than 24 hours of antibiotics is rarely justified. It does not lower infection rates, but can select for more resistant organisms later in the hospital stay.

Second-Generation Cephalosporins

Agents: cefamandole, **cefuroxime**, **cefoxitin**, cefotetan, loracarbef, cefdinir, cefmetazole, cefonicid, cefaclor, **cefprozil**

Compared to first-generation cephalosporins, second-generation agents have better Gram-negative activity and generally weaker Gram-positive activity, though they are still used for these organisms. They are more stable against Gram-negative beta-lactamases and are particularly active against *Haemophilus influenzae* and *Neisseria gonorrhea*. Though the second-generation agents are the most numerous class of cephalosporins, they are probably the least utilized in U.S. hospitals.

Spectrum

Good: some enteric Gram negative rods, *Haemophilus, Neisseria*

Moderate: streptococci, staphylococci, anaerobes (cefotetan, cefoxitin, cefmetazole)

Poor: enterococci, MRSA, *Pseudomonas*

Adverse Effects

Similar to other beta-lactams. Cephalosporins with the *N*-methylthiotetrazole (MTT) side chain—cefamandole, cefmetazole, and cefotetan—can inhibit vitamin K production and prolong bleeding. These MTT cephalosporins can also cause a disulfuram-like reaction when co-administered with ethanol. While most people in the hospital do not have access to alcoholic beverages while being treated for infections, outpatients need to be counseled on this interaction. The interaction is a favorite on board exams.

◼ Important Facts

- Cefoxitin, cefotetan, and cefmetazole are cephamycins. They are grouped with the second-generation cephalosporins because they have similar activity, with one important exception: anaerobes. Cephamycins have activity against many anaerobes in the gastrointestinal tract and cefoxitin and cefotetan are often used for surgical prophylaxis in abdominal surgery.
- Loracarbef is technically a carbacepham. This point is forgettable.
- Cefaclor, cefprozil, and loracarbef are available only orally. Cefuroxime is available in both intravenous and oral formulations, and the others are IV only.
- Like first-generation cephalosporins, second-generation agents do not cross the blood-brain barrier.

What They're Good For

Upper respiratory tract infections, community-acquired pneumonia, gonorrhea, surgical prophylaxis (cefotetan, cefoxitin, cefuroxime).

Don't Forget!

The cephamycins have good intrinsic anaerobic activity but resistance to them is increasing in *Bacteroides fragilis* group infections. When using them for surgical prophylaxis, limit the duration of antibiotic exposure after surgery. If an infection does develop, use alternative agents such as beta-lactamase inhibitor combinations or another Gram-negative agent with metronidazole.

Third-Generation Cephalosporins

Agents: ceftriaxone, **cefotaxime**, **ceftazidime**, **cefpodoxime**, **cefixime**, ceftibuten

Third-generation cephalosporins have greater Gram-negative activity than the first and second generation drugs. They also have good streptococcal activity, but generally lesser staphylococcal activity than previous generations of cephalosporins. These are broad-spectrum agents that have many different uses.

Spectrum

Good: streptococci, enteric Gram-negative rods, *Pseudomonas* (ceftazidime only)

Moderate: MSSA (except ceftazidime)

Poor: enterococci, *Pseudomonas* (except ceftazidime), anaerobes, MRSA

Adverse Effects

Similar to other beta-lactams. Third-generation cephalosporins have been shown to be one of the classes of antibiotics with the strongest association with *Clostridium difficile* associated diarrhea. Cefpodoxime has the MTT side-chain that can inhibit vitamin K production.

■ Important Facts

- Ceftazidime is the exception to the spectrum of activity rule for third-generation agents. Unlike the others, it is antipseudomonal and lacks clinically useful activity against Gram-positive organisms.
- Ceftriaxone, cefotaxime, and ceftazidime cross the blood-brain barrier effectively and are useful for the treatment of CNS infections. However, their differences in spectrum lead clinicians to use them for different types of infections. Ceftazidime would be a poor choice for community-acquired meningitis, where *Streptococcus pneumoniae* predominates.
- Third-generation cephalosporins are notorious for inducing resistance among Gram-negative rods. Though they can be useful in nosocomial infections, too much broad-spectrum utilization can result in harder-to-treat organisms.
- Ceftriaxone has the characteristic of having dual modes of elimination via both renal and biliary excretion. It does not need to be adjusted for renal dysfunction.

What They're Good For

Lower respiratory tract infections, pyelonephritis, nosocomial infections (ceftazidime), Lyme disease (ceftriaxone), meningitis, skin and soft tissue infections, febrile neutropenia (ceftazidime).

Don't Forget!

Ceftriaxone is a once-daily drug for almost all indications *except* meningitis. Make sure your meningitis patients receive the full 2 gram IV q12h dose, and also use vancomycin and ampicillin, if the latter is warranted.

Fourth-Generation Cephalosporins

Agent: cefepime

There is only one fourth-generation cephalosporin, cefepime. Cefepime is the broadest-spectrum cephalosporin, with activity against both Gram-negative organisms including *Pseudomonas* and Gram-positive organisms. One way to remember its spectrum is to think that cefazolin + ceftazidime = cefepime. New cephalosporins with even broader spectra are in development.

Spectrum

Good: MSSA, streptococci, *Pseudomonas*, enteric Gram-negative rods
Moderate: *Acinetobacter*
Poor: enterococci, anaerobes, MRSA

Adverse Effects

Similar to other beta-lactams.

▪ Important Facts

- Cefepime is a broad-spectrum agent. It is a good empiric choice for nosocomial infections, but overkill for many community-acquired infections. Be sure to de-escalate therapy if possible when you empirically treat with cefepime.

- For monotherapy of febrile neutropenia, cefepime is a better choice than ceftazidime due to its better Gram-positive activity. It may also induce less resistance in GNRs than third-generation cephalosporins, but it is still not a good drug to overuse.

What It's Good For

Febrile neutropenia, nosocomial pneumonia, post-neurosurgical meningitis, other nosocomial infections.

Don't Forget!

Cefepime is primarily used for nosocomial infections. Although it is indicated for infections of the urinary tract and lower respiratory tract, it is overkill for most community-acquired sources of these infections.

Carbapenems

Agents: imipenem/cilastatin, meropenem, ertapenem, doripenem

Carbapenems are among our most broad-spectrum antibacterial drugs, particularly imipenem, doripenem, and meropenem. They possess a beta-lactam ring and share the same mechanism of action of beta-lactams, but are structurally unique and differ from both penicillins and cephalosporins. Their broad spectrum makes them both appealing and unappealing for empiric therapy, depending on the infection being treated and the risk factors of the patient for a resistant organism. Imipenem, doripenem, and meropenem have similar spectra of activity; ertapenem has important deficiencies in its spectrum that must be learned.

Spectrum

Good: MSSA, streptococci, anaerobes, enteric Gram-negative rods, *Pseudomonas* (not ertapenem), *Acinetobacter* (not ertapenem), ESBL-producing Gram-negative rods

Moderate: enterococci (not ertapenem)

Poor: MRSA, penicillin-resistant streptococci

Adverse Effects

Similar to other beta-lactams, but with a higher propensity to induce seizures. This is particularly problematic with imipenem. Minimize the risk by calculating appropriate doses for patients with renal dysfunction and avoiding imipenem use in patients with meningitis, because it can cross the blood-brain barrier more readily.

▣ Important Facts

- Imipenem is metabolized in the kidney to a nephrotoxic product. Cilastatin blocks the renal dehydropeptidase that catalyzes this reaction and prevents this metabolism from occurring. It is always co-administered with imipenem for this reason.

- Carbapenems are very broad-spectrum agents. Imipenem, doripenem, and meropenem are particularly broad and should not be used empirically for most community-acquired infections. They are good choices for many types of nosocomial infections, particularly in patients who have received many other classes of antibiotics during their hospital stay.

- Although ertapenem has weaker activity than the other carbapenems for a relatively few organisms, this is significant enough to change the utility of the drug. Ertapenem is a poor choice for many nosocomial infections, particularly nosocomial pneumonia where both *Pseudomonas* and *Acinetobacter* are frequent causes of infection. However, it is administered only once a day and thus more convenient than the other carbapenems, so it may be a better choice for home infusion therapy of susceptible infections.

- Carbapenems can elicit an allergic reaction in patients with a history of penicillin allergy. While it is unknown what percentage of patients with penicillin allergy will react to a carbapenem, one study showed the incidence of such reactions to be as high as 50% with a proven penicillin allergy (keep in mind that many penicillin allergies are unproven). More recent studies have shown this number to be much lower. Nevertheless, take the possibility of cross-reactivity seriously.

What They're Good For

All: mixed aerobic/anaerobic infections, infections caused by ESBL-producing organisms, intra-abdominal infections.

Imipenem, doripenem, meropenem: nosocomial pneumonia, febrile neutropenia, other nosocomial infections.

Don't Forget!

Check your dosing in patients with renal dysfunction to minimize the risk of carbapenem-induced seizures.

Monobactams

Agent: aztreonam

Aztreonam is the only monobactam available. Structurally, aztreonam contains only the four-membered ring of the basic beta-lactam structure, hence the name monobactam. Aztreonam's quirk is that it seems to be safe to administer to patients with allergies to other beta-lactams, except patients who have a specific allergy to ceftazidime. This cross-reactivity seems to be due to the fact that ceftazidime and aztreonam share an identical side chain. Ceftazidime and aztreonam also virtually share the same spectrum of activity. It is reasonably safe to remember the utility of aztreonam by thinking of it as ceftazidime without allergic cross-reactivity with other beta-lactams.

Spectrum
Good: *Pseudomonas*, most Gram-negative rods
Moderate: *Acinetobacter*
Poor: Gram-positive organisms, anaerobes

Adverse Effects
Similar to other beta-lactams, but with a low incidence of hypersensitivity.

▓ Important Facts

- Aztreonam shares a mechanism of action and pharmacodynamic profile with other beta-lactams. Because it is a Gram-negative drug that is often used in patients with penicillin allergies, it is often confused with aminoglycosides. It is chemically unrelated to aminoglycosides and does not share their toxicities.
- Aztreonam is a type of beta-lactam, and combination therapy with it and other beta-lactams against the same organism is unwarranted. Try adding a non-beta-lactam drug to your empiric regimen for serious nosocomial infections instead.

What It's Good For
Gram-negative infections including *Pseudomonas*, particularly in patients with a history of beta-lactam allergy.

Don't Forget!
Before using aztreonam in your patients with beta-lactam allergies, investigate whether the reaction was specifically to ceftazidime. If you cannot determine this and the reaction was anaphylactoid, proceed with caution or use an alternative agent.

Glycopeptides

6

Agent: vancomycin

To date, there are two glycopeptides in clinical use: vancomycin and teicoplanin. Teicoplanin is not used in the United States. At least three more glycopeptides are in late stages of clinical development: oritavancin, dalbavancin, and telavancin. We will limit our discussion to vancomycin.

Vancomycin is invaluable, because it has activity against all things Gram-positive that have not learned to become resistant to it. Many enterococci (especially *E. faecium*) have figured this out and we call them vancomycin-resistant enterococci (VRE). A few staphylococci have learned it from the enterococci, but this is currently very rare. Streptococci are susceptible.

Spectrum

Good: MSSA, MRSA, streptococci, *Clostridium difficile*
Moderate: enterococci
Poor: anything Gram-negative

Adverse Effects

Ototoxicity and nephrotoxicity are adverse effects classically assigned to vancomycin. Although the historical evidence linking these with vancomycin is poor, recent studies have shown that it may be nephrotoxic in high doses. The early formulation of vancomycin was brown, and clinicians trying to amuse themselves dubbed it "Mississippi mud." The current formulation is clear and lacks those potentially toxic excipients. A histamine-mediated reaction called red man syndrome can occur; the patient may feel warm, flushed, and can be hypotensive. It can be prevented by slowing the infusion rate and is not a true allergy. Antihistamines can also ameliorate the reaction.

Dosing Issues

Vancomycin exhibits time-dependent killing, but we often dose it as a concentration-dependent drug (big doses less frequently) for the sake of convenience. It is often pharmacokinetically monitored, but the evidence that these concentrations mean anything is lacking, particularly for peak concentrations. Trough concentrations can be used to ensure that the drug is not being eliminated too quickly, and different indications have different preferred trough ranges.

▦ Important Facts

- Oral vancomycin is absorbed poorly. Its only use is for the treatment of *Clostridium difficile*-associated disease. Also, intravenous vancomycin does not reach intracolonic concentrations high enough to kill *C. difficile*, so oral is the only way to go.
- Do not overreact if your vancomycin trough is too high. Was it drawn correctly? If so, increase your dosing interval.
- Although vancomycin is active against staphylococci, it does not kill MSSA as quickly as beta-lactams. Does your patient have MSSA? Use nafcillin or cefazolin instead.

- Recently, a phenomenon described as "MIC creep" has been seen with staphylococci and vancomycin. MICs have been rising to vancomycin in many institutions, and while they have not yet reached the level of resistance they are increasing within the range labeled as susceptible, that is, ≤2 mcg/ml. However, patients receiving vancomycin for serious infections caused by staphylococci with an MIC = 2 mcg/ml to vancomycin have been shown to have worse outcomes than those with lower MICs. This issue is one that warrants careful attention.

What It's Good For

Vancomycin is a drug of choice for MRSA infections and for empiric use where MRSA is a concern, such as nosocomial pneumonia. It is also useful in other Gram-positive infections when the patient has a severe beta-lactam allergy. Some of the investigational glycopeptides also have activity against vancomycin-resistant organisms.

Don't Forget!

Are you *sure* that trough concentration was drawn correctly?

Fluoroquinolones

7

Agents: ciprofloxacin, levofloxacin, moxifloxacin, gemifloxacin

Many of the fluoroquinolones are near-ideal antibiotics: they have broad-spectrum activity that includes Gram-positive, Gram-negative, and atypical organisms; display excellent oral bioavailability; and have a relatively low incidence of adverse effects. These characteristics have led to overprescribing and the inevitable rise in resistance, despite recommendations to reserve this class. The newer drugs (levo, moxi, gemi) gain increasing Gram-positive (mostly pneumococcal) activity at the expense of some Gram-negative (mostly *Pseudomonas*) activity. Significant differences among the agents are in **bold**.

Spectrum: Ciprofloxacin

Good: enteric Gram-negatives rods, *H. influenzae*

Moderate: *Pseudomonas*, atypicals (*Mycoplasma, Chlamydia, Legionella*)

Poor: staphylococci, *S. pneumoniae*, anaerobes, enterococci

Spectrum: Levofloxacin/Moxifloxacin/ Gemifloxacin

Good: enteric Gram negatives (*E. coli, Proteus, Klebsiella,* etc.), *S. pnuemoniae,* atypicals (*Mycoplasma, Chlamydia, Legionella*), *H. influenzae*

Moderate: Pseudomonas (**levofloxacin only**), MSSA

Poor: anaerobes (**except moxifloxacin**, which has moderate activity), enterococci

Adverse Effects

GI side effects, headache, and photosensitivity are most common. Rare but serious side effects usually occur in patients with underlying conditions: hyper- or hypoglycemia (diabetes), seizures (seizure disorder), prolongation of the QT interval (underlying arrhythmia or proarrhythmic medications). These effects are dose-related, so review dosing in patients with renal dysfunction and the elderly. Arthralgias (uncommonly) and Achilles tendon rupture (very rarely) may occur. Fluoroquinolones also can cause CNS adverse reactions, including dizziness, confusion, and hallucinations. Elderly patients are particularly susceptible to these. Younger patients may develop insomnia.

Because of toxicities seen in juvenile beagle dogs, fluoroquinolones are absolutely contraindicated in pregnant women and relatively contraindicated in children, although experience with use in children suggests they can be used safely.

Dosing Issues

While ciprofloxacin and levofloxacin have activity against *Pseudomonas*, MICs are typically higher than with other susceptible organisms (e.g., *E. coli*). Thus, when using these drugs to treat *Pseudomonas* infections (or if *Pseudomonas* is strongly suspected), give them at higher, anti-pseudomonal doses: 400 mg IV q8h or 750 mg PO q12h for ciprofloxacin; 750 mg IV/PO daily for levofloxacin.

Important Facts

- Bioavailability of all fluoroquinolones is 80–100%, so oral dose = IV dose (**except ciprofloxacin**, PO = 1.25 times IV dose).
- Fluoroquinolones chelate cations and their oral bioavailability is *significantly decreased* when administered with calcium, iron, antacids, milk, or multivitamins. Separate these agents by at least 2 hours or have your patient take a week off of the supplements, if possible. Administration with tube feedings is also problematic.
- Most fluoroquinolones are cleared renally and require dose reduction in renal dysfunction. **Moxifloxacin is the exception** because it is not excreted into the urine it is also not approved for treatment of urinary tract infections. Gemifloxacin has dual elimination, and its utility in treating urinary tract infections is not yet established, though it does require dose adjustment in renal failure.

What They're Good For

Not everything, despite the temptation. Remember, the longer you want to be able to use these drugs, the more restraint should be exercised now. Indications for the fluoroquinolones are listed in Table 7-1.

Don't Forget!

When using the oral forms of fluoroquinolones, be especially careful to avoid co-administering with chelating agents (calcium, magnesium, aluminum, etc.). Also be cautious of using these drugs in patients with conditions or drugs that prolong the QT interval.

TABLE 7-1
Indications for Fluoroquinolones

Indication	Cipro	Levo	Moxi	Gemi
CAP, sinusitis, AECB	−	+	+	+
UTI	+	+	−	?
Intra-abdominal infection	+	+	+	?
Systemic Gram-negative infections	+	+	+	?
Skin/soft tissue infection	−	+	+	+
Single-dose treatment of gonorrhea	+	+	?	?
Pseudomonas infections (+/- beta-lactam)	+	+	−	−
Treatment/prophylaxis in bioterrorism scenarios (active vs. anthrax, plague, tularemia)	+	+	?	?

+ = approved/studied/makes sense for this indication.
? = should work, no clinical data.
− = suboptimal.

Aminoglycosides

8

Agents: gentamicin, tobramycin, amikacin, streptomycin, spectinomycin

The aminoglycosides as a class dispel the notion that antibiotics are largely non-toxic. These drugs have a narrow therapeutic window, and improper dosing carries the risk of inflicting significant toxicity (primarily nephro- and ototoxicity) on your patients. Because of this, there has been a reduction in their use as primary therapy for most infections. That being said, they retain good activity against many problem pathogens (such as *Pseudomonas* and *Acinetobacter*) that have developed resistance to the more benign drug classes. They are also excellent at synergizing with the beta-lactams and glycopeptides to improve the efficiency of bacterial killing. Gentamicin and tobramycin are the most widely used drugs; amikacin is generally reserved for pathogens resistant to the first two; and streptomycin (*Enterococcus*, tuberculosis, and plague) and spectinomycin (gonorrhea) are niche drugs.

Spectrum: Gentamicin/tobramycin/amikacin

Good: Gram-negatives (*E. coli, Klebsiella, Pseudomonas, Acinetobacter*, most others)

Moderate: in combination with a beta-lactam or glycopeptide: staphylococci (including MRSA), viridans streptococci, enterococci

Poor: atypicals, anaerobes, Gram-positive organisms (as monotherapy)

Adverse Effects

Nephrotoxicity: Oliguric acute renal failure, preceded by a rising serum creatinine, is a dose-related adverse effect of aminoglycosides. Risk can be reduced by correct dosing (including the use of extended-interval dosing), as well as avoidance of co-administration of other nephrotoxins (cyclosporin, cisplatin, foscarnet, etc.).

Ototoxicity: Aminoglycosides cause dose-related cochlear and vestibular toxicity. For patients anticipated to receive long-term (>2 weeks) aminoglycosides, baseline audiology is recommended.

Neuromuscular blockade can occur when aminoglycosides are given, particularly in high doses in patients who are receiving therapeutic paralysis.

▉ Important Facts

- Once-daily or extended-interval aminoglycoside dosing leverages the concentration-dependent killing of the drugs to create an equally effective, more convenient, and possibly safer dosing regimen. However, there are many populations in which once-daily dosing has had minimal study, including the pregnant, the critically ill, those with significant renal dysfunction, and the morbidly obese. Use this dosing method with caution, if at all, in these populations.
- Aminoglycoside serum levels can help guide appropriate dosing and reduce the risk of toxic-

ity, but they must be drawn correctly to have meaningful interpretations. For traditional dosing methods, a peak level should be drawn half an hour after the end of the infusion, while trough levels should be drawn within 30 minutes of the next dose. For once-daily dosing there are a number of potential monitoring points, including midpoint and trough levels.

- Aminoglycosides have relatively poor distribution into tissues, including the lungs. They have minimal nervous system penetration. This makes them less than optimal as monotherapy for many severe infections. It also means that a dose should be based on the patient's ideal or adjusted body weight, rather than his or her total body weight. Given the high prevalence of morbid obesity, serious overdosing of patients can occur if the patient's total body weight is used.

What They're Good For

In combination with a beta-lactam agent, treatment of serious infections with documented or suspected Gram-negative pathogens, including febrile neutropenia, sepsis, exacerbations of cystic fibrosis, and ventilator-associated pneumonia. In combination with a beta-lactam or glycopeptide, treatment of serious Gram-positive infections, including endocarditis, osteomyelitis, and sepsis. In combination with other antimycobacterials, treatment of drug-resistant infections with *M. tuberculosis* or other mycobacteria.

Don't Forget!

Most aminoglycoside toxicity is dose-related, so get the dose right from the start by adjusting for renal dysfunction and using ideal or adjusted body weight. Pharmacokinetic concentrations are useful for monitoring and dosing aminoglycosides if they are drawn correctly.

Tetracyclines and Glycylcyclines

9

Agents: doxycycline, minocycline, **tetracycline, tigecycline** (a glycylcycline)

Once considered broad-spectrum antibiotics, the relentless advance of bacterial resistance and the off-patent status of the drugs have reduced the use of tetracyclines to niche indications. They are useful (but not highly studied) alternatives for the treatment of common respiratory tract infections and drugs of choice for a variety of uncommon infections. Doxycycline is preferred in most situations over tetracycline and minocycline. This class may see a revival with the introduction of the glycylcyclines (starting with tigecycline), which evade most tetracycline resistance mechanisms and have a broad spectrum of activity.

Spectrum: Tetracycline/doxycycline/minocycline

Good: atypicals, rickettsia, spirochetes (e.g., *T. pallidum, B. burgdorferi, H. pylori*)

Moderate: staphylococci (including MRSA), *S. pneumoniae, S. pyogenes*

Poor: most Gram-negative rods, anaerobes, enterococci

Spectrum: Tigecycline

Good: atypicals, enterococci (including VRE), staphylococci (including MRSA), *S. pnuemoniae, S. pyogenes*

Acceptable: most Gram-negatives, anaerobes

Poor: Pseudomonas, Proteus, Providencia, Prevotella

Adverse Effects

GI side effects (nausea, diarrhea) and photosensitivity are most common. Tigecycline, although an IV drug, can cause severe nausea, vomiting, and diarrhea. Tetracyclines can cause esophageal irritation, and patients should take the drug with water, while standing up if possible. Minocycline may cause dizziness and vertigo. All tetracyclines can cause discoloration of developing teeth and are contraindicated in pregnant women and children younger than 8 years old.

▋ Important Facts

- Doxycycline and minocycline bioavailability is approximately 100%. Tigecycline is IV only.
- Tetracyclines chelate cations and their oral bioavailability is *decreased significantly* when administered with calcium, iron, antacids, milk, or multivitamins. Separate these agents by at least 2 hours or take a week off of the supplements, if possible. Food decreases the absorption of tetracycline substantially, but minocycline and doxycycline minimally.
- Doxycycline does not need to be adjusted in renal or hepatic dysfunction; tetracycline is eliminated renally and should not be used in cases of renal insufficiency (it can worsen renal dysfunction).

What They're Good For

Uncomplicated respiratory tract infections: acute exacerbations of chronic bronchitis, sinusitis, community-acquired pneumonia. They are the drugs of choice for many tick-borne diseases. Alternative for skin/soft tissue infections, syphilis, pelvic inflammatory disease (with cefoxitin). Alternative to ciprofloxacin in bioterrorism scenarios (active vs. anthrax, plague, tularemia). Malaria prophylaxis and treatment. Tigecycline may have a role in the treatment of complicated polymicrobial infections.

Don't Forget!

Ask patients if they take mineral supplements (like calcium and iron) at home. Just because it is not on their medication profile does not mean they do not take it. Having a patient wash down the doxycycline that you prescribed with a calcium supplement or a glass of milk completely negates the therapeutic plan. Does your patient add milk to their coffee or tea? Even this small amount should be avoided with tetracyclines as well.

Macrolides and Ketolides

10

Agents: erythromycin, **clarithromycin**, **azithromycin**, **telithromycin** (a ketolide)

Macrolides are among the antibiotics used most frequently in the outpatient setting because of their broad coverage of respiratory pathogens. Their coverage is broad, but not particularly deep, as there is increasing resistance to these agents (especially in *Streptococcus pneumoniae)*. To combat this resistance, the ketolide derivatives (including telithromycin) have been introduced with better coverage of resistant *S. pneumoniae*. Unfortunately telithromycin may have more hepatotoxicity than its peers. Although erythromycin is the class patriarch, because of its toxicity, drug interactions, and more limited spectrum, it has little use anymore except as a GI stimulant.

Spectrum: clarithromycin/azithromycin

Good: atypicals, *Haemophilus influenzae, Moraxella catarrhalis, Helicobacter pylori, Mycobacterium avium*

Moderate: S. pneumoniae (telithromycin > macrolides), S. pyogenes

Poor: staphylococci, enteric Gram-negative rods (azithro > clarithro), anaerobes, enterococci

Adverse Effects

Gastrointestinal: Significant GI adverse effects (nausea/vomiting, diarrhea) have been associated with the macrolides. Erythromycin is the worst offender—it is employed as a prokinetic agent for patients with impaired GI motility.

Hepatic: Rare but serious adverse hepatic events have been associated with the macrolides. Recently a number of cases of hepatic failure leading to transplantation and death have been associated with telithromycin use.

Cardiac: Prolongation of the QT interval has been seen with the macrolides, again most commonly with erythromycin. Use with caution in patients with preexisting heart conditions, those on antiarrhythmic drugs, or those taking interacting drugs (see below).

▪ Important Facts

* ***Drug interaction alert!*** These drugs (with the exception of azithromycin) are potent inhibitors of drug-metabolizing cytochrome P450 enzymes. Therefore be sure to screen your patient's regimen with a computerized drug interaction checker or a drug information resource before starting these agents.

* Azithromycin has a prolonged half-life such that a 3–5 day course may be adequate for most infections, instead of 7–10 days with other drugs. This makes use of the Z-pak® and the newer Z-max® possible.

* Macrolides are bacteriostatic drugs and are not appropriate for infections in which cidal activity is usually required (meningitis, endocarditis, osteomyelitis, etc.).

- Prevpac® is a combination of drugs prescribed for eradication of *H. pylori* and the treatment of peptic ulcer disease. In addition to clarithromycin and lansoprazole, it contains amoxicillin. Be sure to screen patients for beta-lactam allergies before administering it.

What They're Good For
Upper and lower respiratory tract infections, chlamydia, atypical mycobacterial infections, and traveler's diarrhea (azithromycin). Clarithromycin is a key component in the treatment of *H. pylori*-induced gastrointestinal ulcer disease in combination with other drugs and acid-suppressive agents.

Don't Forget!
Sure, macrolides are good respiratory tract drugs and relatively benign, but do you really need to be treating this patient's nonspecific (possibly viral) cough and cold with *any* antibiotic? Besides causing possible adverse reactions and wallet toxicity, overuse of these drugs has contributed to increasing resistance. How about some decongestants, acetaminophen, and chicken soup instead?

11

Oxazolidinones

Agent: linezolid

Currently linezolid is the only member of the oxazolidinone class. Linezolid has become a useful (albeit expensive) antibiotic for the treatment of various resistant Gram-positive infections. Its use is likely to increase as MRSA becomes more prevalent in the community, but remember that there are other drugs for these infections as well.

Spectrum

Good: MSSA, MRSA, streptococci (including multi-drug resistant *S. pneumoniae*), enterococci (including VRE), *Nocardia*

Moderate: some atypicals

Poor: all Gram-negatives, anaerobes

Adverse Effects

Linezolid is generally well-tolerated, but can cause bone marrow suppression, particularly thrombocytopenia. This tends to occur after 2 or more weeks of therapy and warrants monitoring. Peripheral neuropathy may occur after even more prolonged therapy (months) due to toxicity to mitochondria.

■ Important Facts

- Linezolid has bioavailability approaching 100% and its oral formulation increases its utility.

- It is also an inhibitor of monoamine oxidase (MAO) and can cause serotonin syndrome when given concurrently with serotonergic agents such as selective serotonin reuptake inhibitors (SSRIs)—avoid concurrent use if possible. Recent evidence has shown this to be uncommon, but it does occur.
- Linezolid doses do not need to be adjusted in cases of renal or hepatic dysfunction.
- Both oral and intravenous formulations are very expensive, but the oral formulation is less expensive than home infusion vancomycin and a nurse.

What It's Good For

Infections caused by resistant Gram-positive organisms such as VRE and MRSA, and nosocomial pneumonia or skin and soft tissue infections.

Don't Forget!

Monitor patients for bone marrow suppression, particularly during long-term therapy with linezolid. Avoid concurrent serotonergic drug use if possible. Remember that many SSRIs have long half-lives, so simply discontinuing SSRI use does not avoid a potential interaction. Monitor patients for signs and symptoms of serotonin syndrome if the interaction cannot be avoided.

12

Nitroimidazoles

Agents: metronidazole, tinidazole

Nitroimidazoles are around to clean up bugs that the big drug classes—penicillins, cephalosporins, fluoroquinolones, macrolides—for the most part miss. Worried about gut anaerobes? Metronidazole is there for you. Thinking about parasites in your patient with diarrhea? Try metronidazole or its new cousin tinidazole, which has a similar spectrum of activity to metronidazole but is only approved for parasitic infections. And of course, if you have gone overboard with the antibiotics and given your patient *C. difficile* colitis, turn to metronidazole as your first-line therapy. Just remember the limitations of these drugs: they do *not* have adequate activity against aerobic bacteria—staphylococci, streptococci, *E. coli,* and such.

Spectrum: metronidazole

Good: Gram-negative and Gram-positive anaerobes, including *Bacteroides*, *Fusobacterium*, and *Clostridium* spp., protozoa including *Trichomonas*, *Entamoeba*, and *Giardia*

Moderate: Helicobacter pylori

Poor: aerobic Gram-negative and Gram-positive organisms, anaerobes that reside in the mouth (*Peptostreptococcus*; *Actinomyces*, *Propionibacterium*)

Adverse Effects

Gastrointestinal: Nausea, vomiting, and diarrhea, along with a metallic taste, are not uncommon with metronidazole. More severe adverse reactions such as hepatitis and pancreatitis are rare.

Neurologic: Dose-related, reversible peripheral neuropathy has occasionally been reported with metronidazole, along with very rare cases of confusion and seizures.

▨ Important Facts

- Metronidazole has a reputation for causing a disulfiram-like reaction with the consumption of alcohol, because of its inhibition of aldehyde dehydrogenase. It is prudent to have patients abstain from alcohol while taking metronidazole. Much more considerable is the interaction with warfarin, whose anticoagulant properties are significantly potentiated by inhibition of warfarin metabolism. Careful monitoring and warfarin dose reduction may be necessary.

- Metronidazole has excellent (~100%) bioavailability and none of the drug-chelating concerns of the fluoroquinolones; thus patients should be switched from IV to oral metronidazole as soon as they are tolerating oral medications.

- Resistance to metronidazole among isolates of *C. difficile* is uncommon, but treatment failure with this infection is not. The organism can exist as an antibiotic-resistant spore and cause relapses after the end of treatment. Retreatment with metronidazole is reasonable in most cases of relapsing *C. difficile*, although treatment with oral vancomycin is an alternative. Other alternatives are being developed for *C. difficile* infection as well.

What They're Good For

Infections with documented or suspected abdominal anaerobic bacteria, with adjunctive coverage of aerobes by a second drug when necessary. Treatment of vaginal trichomoniasis and gastrointestinal infections caused by susceptible protozoa (amebiasis, giardiasis, etc.). Metronidazole is also a component of therapy for *H. pylori* gastrointestinal ulcer disease in combination with other antibacterials and acid-suppressive drugs.

Don't Forget!

The gastrointestinal flora of humans is a delicate ecosystem—disturb it at your patient's peril. Metronidazole's effect on the normal (primarily anaerobic) gastrointestinal flora can set up your patients for colonization with nasty bugs such as VRE; determine whether you really need anaerobic coverage.

13

Nitrofurans

Agent: nitrofurantoin

With the rise in resistance among common urinary tract pathogens (primarily *E. coli*), first among trimethoprim/sulfamethoxazole and lately among the fluoroquinolones, clinicians are left searching for an alternative to treat their patients with uncomplicated UTIs. Nitrofurantoin fits nicely into this niche, with good activity against *E. coli* (>90% in most studies) as well as adequate coverage of other common community-acquired UTI pathogens. However, its utility is limited to infections of the lower urinary tract, because of its pharmacokinetic limitations. Thus, nitrofurantoin should not be used for more severe infections such as pyelonephritis and urosepsis.

Spectrum

Good: E. coli, Staphylococcus saprophyticus
Moderate: Citrobacter, Klebsiella, enterococci
Poor: Pseudomonas, Proteus, Acinetobacter, Serratia

Adverse Effects

Gastrointestinal: Nausea and vomiting are occasionally reported. Taking the drug with food may decrease these effects.

Pulmonary: Nitrofurantoin can cause very rare but serious pulmonary toxicity of two forms. First is an acute pneumonitis manifesting as cough, fever, and dyspnea. This form typically resolves soon after drug discontinuation. A chronic pulmonary fibrosis can occur, most commonly with prolonged nitrofurantoin therapy; recovery of lung function is limited after drug discontinuation.

Peripheral neuropathy may also occur.

▨ Important Facts

- It bears repeating: nitrofurantoin is ineffective for infections outside of the lower urinary tract. The drug requires high concentrations for antimicrobial activity, and these are only reached when it concentrates in the urine. Note this also means that in patients who have significant renal dysfunction (e.g., a creatinine clearance of less than 50 ml/min), there is insufficient accumulation of the drug in the urine for activity.
- Nitrofurantoin comes in two formulations: a crystalline form (Macrodantin®) and a macrocrystalline/monohydrate form (Macrobid®). The former is dosed four times daily, the latter BID. Guess which one patients prefer?

What It's Good For

Treatment of uncomplicated cystitis in patients with adequate renal function. Prophylaxis against recurrent uncomplicated lower UTI.

Don't Forget!

To repeat: do not use this drug in anything but uncomplicated cystitis. Nitrofurantoin use in pyelonephritis or urosepsis is a treatment failure waiting to happen.

Streptogramins

14

Agent: quinupristin/dalfopristin

The increase in resistance to antibiotics among staphylococci and enterococci led to pharmaceutical companies increasing the development of drugs to combat these resistant infections. One of the first of the newer drugs to treat VRE and MRSA infections was quinupristin/dalfopristin. These drugs are two different streptogramins given together in a combined formulation. Though each separate streptogramin is bacteriostatic, when given together they act *syner*gistically to give bacteri*cid*al activity against some Gram-positive cocci, hence the brand name of this drug: Synercid®. Quinupristin/dalfopristin initially enjoyed frequent use, particularly to treat VRE infections, but its use has lessened as other agents have come on the market. Other streptogramins have been developed and are used in animals as growth promoters.

Spectrum

Good: MSSA, MRSA, streptococci, *Enterococcus faecium* including vancomycin-resistant strains

Poor: *Enterococcus faecalis*, anything Gram-negative

Adverse Effects

Quinupristin/dalfopristin can cause phlebitis and ideally should be administered via a central line. It is also associated with a high incidence of myalgias and arthralgias that can limit tolerance to therapy. Quinupristin/dalfopristin also inhibits cytochrome P450 3A4 and clinicians need to be aware of potential drug interactions.

■ Important Facts

- Quinupristin/dalfopristin must be mixed and administered with 5% dextrose in water (D5W) solutions only. When mixed with normal saline, the drug becomes insoluble and can crystallize, even when the line is flushed with saline. Be sure that your patient's nurses know to flush the line with D5W or another saline-free diluent. The drug is not available orally.
- The arthralgias and myalgias associated with quinupristin/dalfopristin are significant and should not be underestimated. It may be possible to decrease the severity of them by decreasing the dose, but this could compromise efficacy.

What It's Good For

Infections caused by *E. faecium* or MRSA in patients not responding to or intolerant of other medications.

Don't Forget!

Quinupristin/dalfopristin is not active against *Enterococcus faecalis*. Between the two most common clinical species of *Enterococcus* (*E. faecalis* and *E. faecium*), *E. faecalis* is more common in most hospitals, but less likely to be resistant to vancomycin. For this reason, quinupristin/dalfopristin is better employed as a definitive therapy than an empiric one for enterococci unless you strongly suspect *E. faecium* infection.

15

Cyclic Lipopeptides

Agent: daptomycin

Daptomycin is the only cyclic lipopeptide that has made its way onto the market. It has a unique mechanism of action and target compared to other antibiotics. Daptomycin binds to the cell membrane of Gram-positive bacteria, weakening it and allowing essential ions to leak out of the organism. This leads to a rapid depolarization of the membrane potential and cessation of needed cell processes, leading to cell death. Interestingly, instead of blowing the bacteria apart as beta-lactams do, daptomycin leaves the dead bacteria intact.

Spectrum

Good: MSSA, MRSA, streptococci
Moderate to Good: enterococci, including VRE
Poor: anything Gram-negative

Adverse Effects

Daptomycin has effects on skeletal muscle that can manifest as muscle pain or weakness, or possibly rhabdomyolysis. To monitor for this effect, creatine kinase (CK) concentrations should be checked weekly while on therapy. This toxicity can be decreased by administering the drug no more than once daily and by adjusting the interval in renal dysfunction. Drug fever is also a possibility.

▨ Important Facts

- Daptomycin is active against many resistant Gram-positive organisms, including VRE and MRSA. It has been proven effective in staphylococcal endocarditis (specifically right-sided endocarditis), an indication that few antibiotics have.
- Resistance to daptomycin is very rare, but it has been reported occasionally. Before using daptomycin for your patient, ensure that the lab tests the isolate for daptomycin susceptibility.
- Though it penetrates lung tissue very well, daptomycin cannot be used to treat pneumonia. Human pulmonary surfactant binds to daptomycin, rendering it inactive. Early trials showed poor outcomes in daptomycin-treated pneumonia patients.

What It's Good For

Skin and soft tissue infections caused by resistant Gram-positive organisms and staphylococcal bacteremia, including right-sided endocarditis. Daptomycin also has utility in enterococcal bacteremia, though it is not indicated or well-studied for this use.

Don't Forget!

Monitor CK concentrations and renal function for patients taking daptomycin, particularly if they are on other drugs toxic to skeletal muscle, like HMG-CoA reductase inhibitors.

Trimethoprim/ Sulfamethoxazole

16

Agents: trimethoprim/sulfamethoxazole (TMP/SMX)

Another originally broad-spectrum drug that has fallen victim to the relentless march of antibiotic resistance, the combination of trimethoprim and sulfamethoxazole is still a drug of choice for a number of indications. Resistance tends to vary considerably by geographic region, so consider your local antibiogram before using TMP/SMX as empiric therapy.

Spectrum

Good: *Staphylococcus aureus* including some MRSA, *H. influenzae, Stenotrophomonas maltophilia, Listeria, Pneumocystis jirovecii* (formerly known as *P. carinii*)

Moderate: enteric Gram-negative rods, *S. pneumoniae, Salmonella, Shigella, Nocardia*

Poor: *Pseudomonas,* enterococci, *S. pyogenes,* anaerobes

Adverse Effects

Dermatologic: TMP/SMX frequently causes rash, most commonly due to the sulfamethoxazole component. Interestingly, rash is much more frequent in HIV/AIDS patients. Although these rashes are usually not severe, life-threatening dermatologic reactions such as toxic epidermal necrolysis and Stevens-Johnson syndrome have been documented.

Hematologic: A primarily dose-dependent bone-marrow suppression can be seen with TMP/SMX, especially at the higher doses used to treat *Pneumocystis* infections.

Renal: Confusingly, TMP/SMX can cause both true and pseudo-renal failure. Crystalluria and acute interstitial nephritis due to the SMX component can lead to acute renal failure; however, the blockade of creatinine secretion by TMP can cause an increase in serum creatinine without a true decline in glomerular filtration rate. TMP can also cause hyperkalemia in a fashion similar to the potassium-sparing diuretics (e.g., triamterene).

▦ Important Facts

- For years, TMP/SMX was considered standard first-line therapy for treatment of acute uncomplicated UTI in women. Recent guidelines suggest, however, that in areas with local resistance rates of >15% to 20% in *E. coli*, an alternative drug (e.g., ciprofloxacin or nitrofurantoin) should be used. This recommendation is somewhat controversial because of the increasing rate of fluoroquinolone resistance. Certainly, at a minimum TMP/SMX should not be used for empiric therapy of complicated UTI (pyelonephritis or urosepsis).

- TMP/SMX comes in a fixed, 1:5 ratio of the two components. Dosing is based on the TMP component. The oral form comes in two strengths: single-strength (80:400 mg TMP:SMX) and double-strength (160:800mg TMP:SMX). TMP/SMX has excellent oral bioavailability, allowing for conversion to oral therapy when patients are tolerating oral medications.

- TMP/SMX has a significant drug interaction with warfarin, leading to higher-than-anticipated prothrombin times. Closely monitor patients who receive both drugs, and remember that when the TMP/SMX is continued, clotting times will return to baseline, possibly necessitating dose changes with warfarin.

- TMP/SMX is fairly insoluble in intravenous solutions, and relatively large volumes of diluent are needed for it to go into solution. Be aware that this fluid may be considerable, particularly for volume-overloaded patients such as those with heart failure.

What They're Good For
Treatment of uncomplicated lower urinary tract infections (in areas with low local resistance). Prophylaxis against recurrent urinary tract infections. Treatment of listerial meningitis. Treatment of and prophylaxis for *Pneumocystis jirovecii* pneumonia. Alternative therapy for bacterial prostatitis. Alternative therapy for typhoid fever. Alternative treatment for methicillin-resistant *Staphylococcus aureus* infections.

Don't Forget!
Patients allergic to TMP/SMX may have cross-reactions to other drugs containing sulfonamide moieties, such as furosemide, sulfadiazine, acetazolamide, hydrochlorothiazide, and glipizide.

17

Lincosamides

Agent: clindamycin

Clindamycin can be considered a mix of vancomycin and metronidazole; it has attributes of each drug, but is not quite as good as either one alone. Clindamycin is an alternative when treatment requires Gram-positive activity (as with beta-lactam allergies) but with more variable activity than vancomycin against pathogens such as MRSA and *S. pyogenes*. Clindamycin also covers many anaerobic organisms, but there is a higher level of resistance among the Gram-negative anaerobes (such as *B. fragilis*) than with metronidazole. Because of these limitations and its tendency to cause GI toxicity, it is best used empirically for non-severe infections of the skin and oral cavity, or as definitive therapy when susceptibilities are known.

Spectrum: clindamycin

Good: many Gram-positive anaerobes

Moderate: *Staphylococcus aureus* including some MRSA, *Streptococcus pyogenes,* Gram-negative anaerobes, *Chlamydia trachomatis, P. jirovecii, Actinomyces, Toxoplasma*

Poor: enterococci, *Clostridium difficile,* Gram-negative aerobes

Adverse Effects

Gastrointestinal: Diarrhea is one of the most common adverse effects associated with clindamycin. Clindamycin itself can cause relatively benign, self-limiting diarrhea or can result in more severe diarrhea resulting from superinfection with *Clostridium difficile*. *C. difficile*-associated diarrhea and colitis can occur during or after clindamycin therapy and can be life-threatening. Patients with diarrhea need evaluation for *C. difficile* disease, especially if it is severe, associated with fever, or persists after the end of clindamycin therapy.

Dermatologic: Rash may occur with clindamycin, very rarely with severe manifestations such as Stevens-Johnson syndrome.

▮ Important Facts

• Clindamycin is a reasonable alternative drug for the treatment of staphylococcal infections; however, care must be taken in interpreting the antibiotic susceptibility of these isolates. A significant proportion of organisms that are reported as clindamycin-susceptible but erythromycin-resistant may harbor a gene for resistance that may lead to high-level clindamycin resistance during therapy. Erythromycin-resistant, clindamycin-susceptible strains should be screened with a D test (the microbiology lab will know what you mean) before using clindamycin.

• Clindamycin's inhibition of protein synthesis and activity against organisms in stationary-phase growth has been utilized in the treatment of necrotizing fasciitis and other toxin-mediated diseases. Consider the addition of clindamycin to beta-lactam based therapy when treating these types of infections.

What It's Good For

Treatment of skin and soft-tissue infections, infections of the oral cavity, anaerobic intra-abdominal infections. Topically used in the treatment of acne. Clindamycin is a second-line agent (in combination with primaquine) in the treatment of *P. jirovecii* pneumonia. It is also used to treat falciparum malaria in combination with other drugs, to treat bacterial vaginosis, and in the prophylaxis of bacterial endocarditis.

Don't Forget!

Almost all antibiotics have been associated with an increased risk of *C. difficile* disease; however some studies suggest that clindamycin may confer an especially high risk (note that this is a popular board-type question). Although it is a convenient and relatively well-tolerated drug, clindamycin should not be used lightly because of this risk.

PART 3

Antifungal Drugs

Antifungal Drugs

18

Introduction to Antifungal Drugs

Fungi rule their own kingdom. There are thousands of species of these saprophytic and parasitic organisms, but, as with bacteria, only a small minority are pathogens. Most pathogenic fungi are opportunistic and require a compromised host or barrier in order to cause infection in humans. As medical advances in transplantation, oncology, rheumatology, neonatology, geriatrics, and other fields create more hosts for fungi, the practice of medical mycology has expanded greatly.

Fungi exist in two basic forms: yeasts and moulds. Table 18-1 highlights some of the medically important fungi. Yeasts are solitary forms of fungi that reproduce by budding. When they are left to grow in colonies, they have a moist, shiny appearance. Moulds are multi-cellular fungi that consist of many branching hyphae and can reproduce either by translocation of existing hyphae to a new area, or through spore formation and spread. They have a familiar fuzzy appearance, such as the *Rhizopus* that you undoubtedly have seen on bread. In addition to these two basic forms, there are dimorphic fungi that can exist in either form. These fungi are often mould-like at room temperature, but yeast-like at body temperature. They are also called endemic fungi, because they cause infections

TABLE 18-1
Common Clinical Fungi

Yeasts	Dimorphic Fungi	Moulds
Cryptococcus	Histoplasma	Aspergillus
Candida	Blastomyces	Fusarium
	Coccidioides	Scedosporium
	Paracoccidioides	Zygomycetes

endemic to certain regions of the world, such as *Coccidioides immitis*, which causes an infection in the southwestern United States and central California that is sometimes called valley fever.

Yeasts, particularly *Candida* species, have become the fourth leading cause of nosocomial bloodstream infections. This makes them important infectious agents that are worthy of our attention. Unfortunately, specific diagnostic criteria for invasive *Candida* infections are lacking. Moulds generally only cause invasive disease in immunocompromised hosts, but should be considered in patients with various levels of immune system suppression, not just those in the most severe category. Dimorphic fungi usually cause mild, self-limited disease, but some can also cause fatal disseminated disease, particularly in patients with suppressed immunity.

There are several problems with antifungal pharmacotherapy that often make treating fungal infections more difficult than treating bacterial infections. One reason is that fungal disease often presents no differently than bacterial disease but the pathogens can be more difficult to isolate on culture. This makes the prompt initiation of empiric therapy important when invasive fungal infections are suspected. Prophylaxis is also used in highly susceptible populations to prevent fungal in-

fections from developing. Another concern with the
treatment of fungal disease is that most centers do
not conduct antifungal susceptibility testing. This
forces clinicians to guess at likely susceptibility
patterns based on speciation rather than true test
results. Further, the capabilities of the host significantly affect the likelihood of success in treating an
invasive fungal infection. For neutropenic patients
with mycoses, neutrophil recovery is a significant
predictor of success, and patients with a prolonged
immunocompromised status have a much worse
prognosis. Therefore, while the selection of an appropriate antifungal is important, control of patient risk factors for fungal infection are perhaps
more so, whether it is the need to remove a central
venous catheter or to decrease doses of immunosuppressants.

Unlike the abundance of drugs available to kill
bacteria, the number of systemic antifungal drugs
is much lower. Selective toxicity is more difficult to
achieve with eukaryotic fungi than with prokary-
otic bacteria. Recently, several newly marketed
agents have changed the way fungal infections are
treated. The chapters that follow introduce these
agents in more detail.

Polyenes

19

Agents: amphotericin B, lipid formulations of amphotericin B, nystatin (topical)

For many years, amphotericin B deoxycholate was the standard of care for many systemic fungal infections, both for its broad antifungal spectrum and a lack of available alternatives. Polyenes work by binding to ergosterol in the cell membrane of fungi, disrupting its membrane. Amphotericin B is notable for its toxicities, principally nephrotoxicity and infusion-related reactions. To attenuate these toxicities, three lipid forms were developed: amphotericin B colloidal dispersion (ABCD), amphotericin B lipid complex (ABLC), and liposomal amphotericin B (LAmB).

Amphotericin B formulations have seen considerably less use since the introduction of the echinocandins and broad-spectrum azoles, but they still have utility. Activity against yeasts and many moulds, proven efficacy in under-studied disease states, and a long history of use helps maintain their place in the antifungal armamentarium.

Spectrum

Good: most species of *Candida* and *Aspergillus*, *Cryptococcus neoformans,* dimorphic fungi, many moulds

Moderate: Zygomycetes
Poor: Candida lusitaniae

Adverse Effects

Nephrotoxicity and infusion-related reactions are the most common adverse effects. Both direct effects on the distal tubule and indirect effects through vasoconstriction of the afferent arteriole cause the nephrotoxicity, and nephrotoxicity also leads to wasting of magnesium and potassium, which thus need supplementation. The infusion-related reactions include fever, chills, and rigors and can be impressive. Less common adverse effects include increased transaminases and rash.

Dosing Issues

The multiple formulations of amphotericin B can lead to confusion over their dosing. Amphotericin B deoxycholate is generally dosed between 0.5–1.5 mg/kg/day, where the lipid formulations are dosed at 3–6 mg/kg/day. Whether the lipid formulations are equivalent is a matter of debate, but most clinicians dose them as if they are. Fatal overdoses of amphotericin B deoxycholate have been given when dosed as the lipid forms are—generally a 5× overdose. Mind your formulation.

▇ Important Facts

- Amphotericin B nephrotoxicity can be attenuated by the process of sodium loading: administered boluses of normal saline before and after the amphotericin infusion. This is an inexpensive and easy way of protecting kidneys.
- Many practitioners administer drugs such as acetaminophen, diphenhydramine, and hydrocortisone to decrease the incidence and severity of infusion-related reactions of amphotericin B.

Meperidine is often given to treat rigors when they develop, but be wary of using this drug in patients who develop renal dysfunction, because it has a neurotoxic metabolite that is eliminated renally.

- Whether differences in efficacy exist between the lipid formulations of amphotericin B is a matter of debate, but differences in safety do exist. In terms of infusion-related reactions, ABCD seems to have the worst while LAmB has the least. All of them have less nephrotoxicity than amphotericin B deoxycholate, but LAmB seems to have the least of all.

- Nystatin is only used topically due to poor tolerance when given systemically.

What They're Good For
Amphotericin B formulations remain the drugs of choice for cryptococcal meningitis and serious forms of some other fungal infections, such as dimorphic fungi and some mould infections. Because of their broad spectrum, they are also a reasonable choice if fungal infection is suspected but the infecting organism is not known. Their use in candidiasis and aspergillosis has declined with the availability of newer, safer agents.

Don't Forget!
Double-check that dose of amphotericin B; which formulation are you using?

Antimetabolites

20

Agent: flucytosine (5-FC)

Flucytosine has a mechanism of action that is distinct from other antifungals in that it has an antimetabolite that interferes with DNA synthesis. Flucytosine was originally investigated as an oncology drug, but was found to be significantly more active against fungi than human cancer cells. The primary role of flucytosine is in combination therapy with amphotericin B formulations for cryptococcal disease. Because of its toxicity and relative lack of efficacy it is rarely used for other infections.

Spectrum

Good: in combination with amphotericin: *Cryptococcus neoformans*, most species of *Candida*

Moderate: monotherapy: *Cryptococcus neoformans*, most species of *Candida*

Poor: moulds, *Candida krusei*

Adverse Effects

Flucytosine, which is also called 5-FC, is fluorouracil (5-FU) for fungi. When this fact is considered, the adverse effects are predictable. Flucytosine is only relatively selective for fungi and can cause considerable bone marrow suppression, particularly in higher doses or during prolonged courses. Gastrointestinal issues are more common complaints, but they are less severe.

Dosing Issues

Flucytosine dosing has evolved from higher doses to lower doses in the combination treatment of crpytococcal disease in an attempt to minimize toxicity. Most drug references quote a daily dosing range of 50–150 mg/kg divided 4 times daily, but many clinicians aim for the low end of this range.

Important Facts

- Drug concentration monitoring is available for flucytosine: check a peak concentration about two hours after the dose is given. However, do not rely on flucytosine concentrations alone to monitor for toxicity—hematology values are more important than drug levels.
- Flucytosine generally should not be used as monotherapy for invasive candidiasis due to the potential emergence of resistance *in vivo*.
- The most common use for flucytosine is in combination with an amphotericin B formulation for cryptococcal meningitis. Though this combination is recommended in guidelines and very common, some clinicians question the value of flucytosine. In the main clinical study for this indication, flucytosine use was associated with more rapid sterility of CSF cultures but no obvious clinical benefit.

What It's Good For

As stated above, the majority of flucytosine use is in the treatment of cryptococcal meningitis in combination with an amphotericin B formulation. It may also be used in other forms of cryptococcal infection and, uncommonly, in *Candida* infection. It may be an acceptable option for the clearance of candiduria in patients who cannot receive fluconazole due to allergy or resistance, but the number of patients who require this therapy is small.

Don't Forget!

Follow your patient's cell counts closely and reconsider the value of flucytosine therapy if hematologic toxicity develops.

Azoles

21

■ Introduction to Azoles

Agents: ketoconazole, **fluconazole**, **itraconazole**, **voriconazole**, **posaconazole**, multiple topical formulations

The azoles are a broad class of antifungal agents whose drug development has recently been expanding. They work by inhibiting fungal cytochrome P450, decreasing ergosterol production. One might expect that this mechanism of action would lead to issues with drug interactions, and this is indeed a significant problem with these drugs.

Azoles have become mainstays of antifungal pharmacotherapy. As they have been developed, agents of variable antifungal spectrums and toxicity profiles have been introduced. These differences are fundamental and are among the most important characteristics to know if you use them clinically. Because they are so different, we will discuss the commonly used systemic agents individually.

Fluconazole

The introduction of fluconazole in 1990 was a break-through in antifungal pharmacotherapy. Fluconazole is highly bioavailable, available in both oral and intravenous formulations, and highly active against many species of *Candida*. Before this, clinicians were faced with the toxicity and inconvenience of amphotericin B for serious forms of candidiasis. It has a low incidence of serious adverse reactions, and converting from intravenous to oral therapy is simple. Though a shift toward non-albicans species of *Candida* has affected the use of fluconazole, it remains an important, frequently utilized agent.

Spectrum

Good: Candida albicans, Candida tropicalis, Candida parapsilosis, Candida lusitaniae, Cryptococcus neoformans, Coccidioides immitis

Moderate: Candida glabrata (can be susceptible dose-dependent, or resistant)

Poor: moulds, many dimorphic fungi, *Candida krusei*

Adverse Effects

Though fluconazole is generally well-tolerated, it can cause hepatotoxicity or rash. It has a lower propensity for serious drug interaction than many other azoles, but interactions still occur with many drugs metabolized by the cytochrome P450 system. QTc prolongation is also possible.

Dosing Issues

Fluconazole doses for systemic fungal infections have been escalated, particularly for the treatment of *Candida glabrata*. Be sure to adjust dosing with regard to renal function, as the drug is eliminated this way. Vulvovaginal candidiasis requires only a one-time dose of 150 mg of fluconazole.

Important Facts

- Fluconazole is poorly active against all *Candida krusei* and some *Candida glabrata*. If you are using it for the latter infection, it is best to check susceptibilities and give 800 mg per day of fluconazole. If your lab does not do susceptibility testing of fungi, try an alternative agent such as an echinocandin.
- Fluconazole is often given as prophylaxis for *Candida* infections in susceptible populations like intensive care unit patients. Are you treating a patient who was receiving it and now has yeast in the blood? Try an echinocandin instead.
- The high bioavailability of fluconazole makes it an excellent therapy to transition to as patients tolerate oral medications.

What It's Good For

Fluconazole remains a drug of choice for many susceptible fungal infections, including invasive and non-invasive candidiasis and cryptococcal disease.

Don't Forget!

Not all species of *Candida* are fluconazole-susceptible. Ensure that you check your patient's isolate before committing to a course of definitive therapy with it.

Itraconazole

Itraconazole is a broader-spectrum azole than fluconazole that could probably have a bigger place in antifungal pharmacotherapy today if it were not for pharmacokinetic issues that have hampered its greater use. It has activity against *Aspergillus* and other mould species and was once commonly used as a step-down therapy in aspergillosis, but this use has declined since voriconazole became available.

Spectrum

Good: *Candida albicans, Candida tropicalis, Candida parapsilosis, Candida lusitaniae, Cryptococcus neoformans, Aspergillus* species, many dimorphic fungi

Poor: *Candida glabrata* and *Candida krusei* (can be susceptible dose-dependent, or resistant), Zygomycetes, many other moulds

Adverse Effects

Itraconazole's adverse effect profile causes more concerns than that of fluconazole. In addition to hepatotoxicity, itraconazole is a negative ionotrope and is contraindicated in patients with heart failure. The oral solution is associated with diarrhea. It is also a stronger inhibitor of cytochrome P450 enzymes and has a long list of drug interactions. QTc prolongation can also occur.

■ **Important Facts**

- Itraconazole comes in two different formulations with different bioavailabilities and requirements. The capsules have lower bioavailability than the solution and are less-preferred for systemic fungal infections.
- The oral formulations of itraconazole have different instructions with regard to taking them with meals. Capsules should always be taken with a full meal, whereas the solution should be taken on an empty stomach. Absorption can also be lowered by agents that decrease gastric acidity, such as proton-pump inhibitors; try having your patients take their itraconazole with a soda.
- Because itraconazole absorption is so erratic and unpredictable, concentrations are often monitored. Consider checking a trough concentration on your patient if he or she is taking it for a serious fungal infection and/or for a long time.

What It's Good For

Itraconazole remains a drug of choice for some dimorphic fungal infections, like histoplasmosis. It once had a bigger role in the management and prophylaxis of aspergillosis and other mould infections, but it has been largely replaced by voriconazole.

Don't Forget!

Watch for those drug interactions, and be sure to counsel your patients on how to take their itraconazole formulation.

Voriconazole

The introduction of voriconazole represented a significant improvement in the treatment of mould infections. It is also a broad-spectrum antifungal like itraconazole, with good activity against *Candida* species and many moulds. Unlike itraconazole, voriconazole is well-absorbed and available in both highly bioavailable oral formulations and an intravenous admixture. Perhaps most importantly, voriconazole was shown to be superior to amphotericin B deoxycholate for invasive aspergillosis and has become the drug of choice for that disease.

Spectrum

Good: *Candida albicans, Candida lusitaniae, Candida parapsilosis, Candida tropicalis, Crytococcus neoformans, Aspergillus* species, many other moulds

Moderate: *Candida glabrata, Candida krusei, Candida albicans* that are fluconazole-resistant, *Fusarium* species

Poor: Zygomycetes

Adverse Effects

In addition to the hepatotoxicity, rash, and drug interactions that are common with this class, voriconazole has some agent-specific adverse effects worth watching. Visual effects such as seeing wavy lines or flashing are very common and dose-related; they tend to go away with continued use. Visual hallucinations can also occur but are less common.

Dosing Issues

Voriconazole has highly variable interpatient pharmacokinetics and non-linear elimination, making it difficult to dose correctly. Some centers monitor voriconazole concentrations, but this test is not yet widely available. If you are treating your patient for a long period of time or are worried about toxicity, consider checking one.

▮ Important Facts

- Voriconazole is active against many fluconazole-resistant strains of *Candida albicans*, but is less active against them than fluconazole-susceptible strains. An echinocandin is a better choice, but consider susceptibility testing if you need to use voriconazole for an oral option.

- Voriconazole is a potent inhibitor of the cytochrome P450 system and the list of drugs that interact with voriconazole is long and varied. Some of them are contraindicated, such as sirolimus, while others, such as calcineurin inhibitors (e.g., cyclosporine), require dose adjustments. This is significant, because many of the patients who require voriconazole are immunosuppressed.

- The intravenous form of voriconazole contains a cyclodextrin vehicle that accumulates in renal dysfunction and may be nephrotoxic. It is contraindicated with a creatinine clearance of less than 50 ml/min. The oral formulations avoid this issue.

- Voriconazole is eliminated hepatically and is unlikely to be useful in the treatment of candiduria.

What It's Good For

Voriconazole is the drug of choice for invasive aspergillosis and is frequently used in the treatment of infections caused by other moulds. It can be used for candidiasis as well, but fluconazole and echinocandins are more frequently used for these infections. Some clinicians use voriconazole in the empiric treatment of febrile neutropenia.

Don't Forget!

Watch for drug interactions with voriconazole, and consider checking drug concentrations if you are using it for an extended course of therapy.

Posaconazole

Posaconazole is the most recently introduced extended-spectrum azole. It is an analog of itraconazole that is substantially more active against many fungi. Currently, it is only indicated for the prophylaxis of fungal infections in neutropenic patients and the treatment of oropharyngeal candidiasis. It is unique amongst the azoles in that it has good activity against the Zygomycetes, a difficult-to-treat class of moulds that most antifungals (voriconazole included) do not treat.

Spectrum

Good: Candida albicans, Candida lusitaniae, Candida parapsilosis, Candida tropicalis, Candida krusei, Aspergillus species, Zygomycetes, many other moulds, dimorphic fungi

Moderate: Fusarium species, Candida glabrata

Though posaconazole is active against these organisms, clinical data are lacking for many of them.

Adverse Reactions

Posaconazole seems to be well-tolerated, though it can cause hepatotoxicity, nausea, and rash. It has the same propensity to cause drug interactions via cytochrome P450 as the other azoles. We will learn more about the adverse effect spectrum of posaconazole as clinical experience with it grows.

Dosing Issues

Posaconazole is only available as an oral suspension. It should always be administered with food to increase its absorption; foods with a high fat concentration improve absorption the most. An intravenous formulation is in development.

▪ Important Facts

- Posaconazole's primary use is in the prophylaxis of fungal infections in high-risk patients. As with voriconazole, many of these patients are taking immunosuppressants that interact with posaconazole, so keep close tabs on those drug concentrations.
- Clinical data with posaconazole for Zygomycete infections is growing, and it is emerging as a drug of choice for these infections.

What It's Good For

Most evidence with posaconazole is with the prophylaxis of fungal infections in susceptible hosts, but it can also be used in zygomycosis, oropharyngeal candidiasis, and fungal infections refractory to other agents.

Don't Forget!

Have your patients take posaconazole with meals to ensure adequate absorption. This is not always possible with neutropenic patients with mucositis.

22

Echinocandins

Agents: caspofungin, micafungin, anidulafungin

The echinocandins are the latest class of antifungal agents to be introduced to clinical practice and are slowly changing the way some fungal diseases are treated. They work by inhibiting the synthesis of beta-1,3-glucan, a component of the fungal cell wall. This mechanism of action is distinct from other antifungals and gives clinicians a new area of fungi to target. The three available echinocandins are similar drugs with virtually indistinguishable spectra. They are very well tolerated and have excellent activity against *Candida*, but suffer from the same pharmacokinetic setback: a lack of an oral formulation. They have considerably fewer drug interactions than azoles, are safer than polyenes, and have great activity against fluconazole-resistant yeasts.

Spectrum

Good: *Candida albicans, Candida glabrata, Candida lusitaniae, Candida parapsilosis, Candida tropicalis, Candida krusei, Aspergillus* species

Moderate: *Candida parapsilosis,* some dimorphic fungi

Poor: Zygomycetes and most non-*Aspergillus* moulds, *Cryptococcus neoformans*

Adverse Effects

Echinocandins have an excellent safety profile. They can cause mild histamine-mediated infusion-related reactions, but these are not common and can be ameliorated by slowing the infusion rate. Hepatotoxicity is also possible with any of these agents; it may be increased with caspofungin when it is co-administered with cyclosporine, but this is still not common.

■ Important Facts

- Differences among the echinocandins are minor and mostly pharmacokinetic. Caspofungin and micafungin are eliminated hepatically by non-cytochrome P450 metabolism, while anidulafungin degrades in the plasma and avoids hepatic metabolism. Despite this unique method of elimination, it is not completely devoid of hepatoxicity.

- Echinocandins have excellent fungicidal activity against *Candida*, but against *Aspergillus* species they exhibit activity that is neither classically cidal nor static. Instead, they cause aberrant, non-functional hyphae to be formed by the actively growing mould.

- All of the echinocandins are less active against *Candida parapsilosis* than the other common clinical species. It has yet to be determined whether this is likely to result in clinical failure, because this organism has been successfully treated with these drugs. If your patient is infected with this organism, be sure to change any intravenous catheters your patient has and consider fluconazole therapy instead.

- Though drug interactions with the echinocandins are minor, there are some of which you should be wary, particularly with caspofungin and micafungin. Be careful when you use them with the immunosuppressants cyclosporine (caspofungin) and sirolimus (micafungin).

What They're Good For

Echinocandins are becoming drugs of choice for invasive candidiasis, particularly in patients who are clinically unstable. They are also useful in the treatment of invasive aspergillosis but do not have the level of supporting data that voriconazole and the polyenes do for this indication. All of them are used for esophageal candidiasis, and some are used in prophylaxis or empiric therapy of fungal infections in neutropenic patients.

Don't Forget!

Echinocandins are great drugs for invasive candidiasis, but they are not cheap. After beginning empiric therapy with an echinocandin, transition your patient to fluconazole if he or she has a susceptible strain of *Candida*.

Selected Normal Human Flora

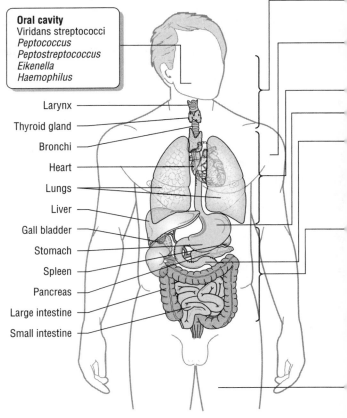

Oral cavity
Viridans streptococci
Peptococcus
Peptostreptococcus
Eikenella
Haemophilus

Larynx

Thyroid gland

Bronchi

Heart

Lungs

Liver

Gall bladder

Stomach

Spleen

Pancreas

Large intestine

Small intestine

Skin
S. epidermidis
S. aureus
Corynebacterium
Propionibacterium

Upper airways
S. pneumoniae
S. pyogenes
Neisseria sp.
H. influenzae
± *S. aureus* (nose)

Stomach
± *H. pylori*

Lower airway:
Normally sterile

**Large intestine
and rectum**
Bacteroides
Fusobacterium
Bifidobacterium
Clostridium
Enterococcus
Lactobacillus
S. bovis
Coliforms
  – *E. coli*
  – *Enterobacter*
  – *Citrobacter*

**Small intestine
Proximal**
  – *Lactobacillus*
  – *Enterococcus*
Distal
  – *Lactobacillus*
  – *Enterococcus*
  – *Bacteroides*
  – Coliforms

Everywhere
S. epidermidis
Corynebacterium

*Genitourinary tract
Lactobacillus   *Corynebacterium*
Streptococcus   *Candida*
E. coli
*In the urinary tract, only the anterior urethra should
be colonized

Clinically Useful Spectra of Activity

	MSSA	MRSA	Strep	Enterococci	GNR	Pseudo	Anaerobes*	Atypicals
Penicillin G			‡	+				
Piperacillin			‡	+	+			
Amp/Sulb	+		‡	‡	+		‡	
Pip/Tazo	‡		‡	‡	‡	‡	‡	
Cefazolin	‡		‡		+			
Cefuroxime	+		+		‡			
Cefotetan	+		+		‡			
Ceftriaxone	+		‡		‡		‡	
Ceftazidime					‡	‡		
Cefepime	+		‡		‡	‡		
Aztreonam					‡	‡		
Imipenem	‡		‡	+	‡	‡	‡	
Ertapenem	‡		‡		‡		‡	
Gentamicin	+(synt)		+(synt)	+(synt)	‡	‡		
Ciprofloxacin	+/-				‡	‡		+
Levofloxacin	‡		‡	+/-	‡	‡		‡
Moxifloxacin	‡		‡	+/-	‡		‡	‡
Doxycycline	+	+/-	+	+/-	+			‡
Tigecycline	‡	‡	‡	‡	‡		‡	‡
Clindamycin	‡	+/-	‡				‡	‡

Vancomycin	++	++	++	++			++	
Azithromycin	+		+		+		+	++
Metronidazole							++	
Telithromycin	+		++				+	++
Daptomycin	++	++	++					
Linezolid	++	++	++	++				+
Quin/Dalf	++	++	++	++				
Nitrofurantoin	+/-		+	+	+		+	
TMP/SMX	++	+/-	+	+	+		+	

Key: ++ = good activity; + = some activity; +/- = variable activity

*Anaerobes here include GI anaerobes except *Clostridium difficile*, for which the only antibiotics with good clinical activity on this list are vancomycin and metronidazole.

†Aminoglycosides have synergistic activity versus Gram-positive cocci only when paired with a cell-wall active agent (e.g., beta-lactams, vancomycin).

MSSA = methicillin-sensitive *Staphylococcus aureus*

MRSA = methicillin-resistant *Staphylococcus aureus*

Strep = streptococci

GNR = aerobic Gram-negative rods (in general, and not including *P. aeruginosa*)

Pseudo = *Pseudomonas aeruginosa*

Amp/sulb = ampicillin/sulbactam

Pip/tazo = piperacillin/tazobactam

Quin/dalf = Quinupristin/dalfopristin

TMP/SMX = trimethoprim/sulfamethoxazole

Index

139